ADAM'S HEART

ADAM'S HEART

◆

An inspiring story about one man's fight against heart disease

Adam Robinson

iUniverse, Inc.
New York Lincoln Shanghai

ADAM'S HEART

An inspiring story about one man's fight against heart disease

iUniverse books may be ordered through booksellers or by contacting:

iUniverse
2021 Pine Lake Road, Suite 100
Lincoln, NE 68512
www.iuniverse.com
1-800-Authors (1-800-288-4677)

ISBN-13: 978-0-595-35634-8 (pbk)
ISBN-13: 978-0-595-80109-1 (ebk)
ISBN-10: 0-595-35634-6 (pbk)
ISBN-10: 0-595-80109-9 (ebk)

Printed in the United States of America

Contents

Introduction

I wrote this book so that I might answer some questions of what life is like after twenty-five years of heart disease—questions that you and your family will have.

The younger days of my childhood gave me the strength to endure and overcome the ongoing battle I face each day with heart disease.

Greasy Creek was a place where family, friends, and neighbors knew and loved each other. It was a place of strength, hard work, and hardship.

As a young man at the age of twenty-nine I had open-heart surgery to replace the aortic valve.

During and after surgery I was scared. I had a lot of questions. What would I be like in ten or twenty years? Would I be alive or dead? Would I be working or on disability?

For ten years after surgery, I lived in fear of what could happen. That fear became an excuse to be disabled, to get fat, to live in pain, to have others feel sorry for me.

Then I realized that I was my own worst enemy. My life had to change. I convinced myself that if my heart was capable of working just fine with my body being thirty-five pounds overweight what would my heart, what would I be capable of if I lost the weight. That thought erased the fear.

At age fifty I have lost the weight by creating my own diet program. I live pain-free because I lost the weight. I have become physically fit by figuring out what exercise I enjoy doing.

I enjoy mountain biking, road biking, flying fishing and I work as a maintenance man. My family and friends forget that I have heart disease.

Contents

Introduction

I wrote this book so that I might answer some questions of what life is like after twenty-five years of heart disease—questions that you and your family will have.

The younger days of my childhood gave me the strength to endure and overcome the ongoing battle I face each day with heart disease.

Greasy Creek was a place where family, friends, and neighbors knew and loved each other. It was a place of strength, hard work, and hardship.

As a young man at the age of twenty-nine I had open-heart surgery to replace the aortic valve.

During and after surgery I was scared. I had a lot of questions. What would I be like in ten or twenty years? Would I be alive or dead? Would I be working or on disability?

For ten years after surgery, I lived in fear of what could happen. That fear became an excuse to be disabled, to get fat, to live in pain, to have others feel sorry for me.

Then I realized that I was my own worst enemy. My life had to change. I convinced myself that if my heart was capable of working just fine with my body being thirty-five pounds overweight what would my heart, what would I be capable of if I lost the weight. That thought erased the fear.

At age fifty I have lost the weight by creating my own diet program. I live pain-free because I lost the weight. I have become physically fit by figuring out what exercise I enjoy doing.

I enjoy mountain biking, road biking, flying fishing and I work as a maintenance man. My family and friends forget that I have heart disease.

MY YOUNGER DAYS

During those golden days of my childhood, I thought, at the time, life was so difficult. Now, with each day that I grow older, my mind often wanders back to precious moments of my youth. At the age of ten, I would have been known as a professional fisherman among all ten year old fishermen in my hollow, so my mother said. As I lay in bed at night, I would listen for rain to hit the roof of the house. I knew if it rained, the small stream in front of my home would turn muddy from the rising water, and the fishing would be good. If rain came on Friday night, it was as if I had just gotten a new toy. For me it was very exciting. Friday was a very special day of the week.

My school sat in the fork of the road. The school was L-shaped with three rooms. The first room was grades one through four. That room was connected to the right-fork road. Grades five through eight were close to the left-fork road. The lunchroom was in the middle. That made the front yard, between the roads and school a diamond shaped playground.

School was a great place! My school had an enrollment of about forty-five kids. When school began in early fall, it was time to play softball. We would show up about one hour early each morning, including our teacher, Mr. Harris Ramey. Mr. Ramey taught grades fifth through eighth. Mr. Booth taught grades one through four. I don't remember Mr. Booth very well. He would only show up to teach classes and never participated in any activities. He left when the last class was finished.

Mr. Ramey was in charge of the school. Class would begin anywhere between 8:30 and 9:00 a.m., just according to how the ballgame was going. Anyone that wasn't playing ball could have been playing volleyball to the right of the ball field. The building that held the lower grades was built about six feet off the ground on concrete posts, which left room underneath for the younger kids to play jump rope, hopscotch or marbles (which was my favorite). If I didn't play marbles, I would play softball. We all would enjoy ourselves until we saw Mr. Ramey walking toward his classroom. Then everyone on the playground would stand silently waiting until Mr. Ramey walked up the two steps, stood on the four by four platform in front of his class and hollered, "Books!" Then we knew it was time for class.

Each teacher would stand on the ground in front of his room. All the kids would line up in front of him. When we were in position, we were asked to turn and face the American flag that stood on an old hickory pole in front of the lunchroom. Once we finished saying the Pledge of Allegiance, we entered our classroom to begin our day.

Our classroom was about thirty feet wide and forty feet long. As we entered the room, the first thing we saw was the teacher's desk. It was a large wooden desk with drawers on each side, accompanied by a wooden chair that the teacher used. The floor was a wooden floor without a finish, and the desk, chair and floor were worn and beaten from years of use. Behind the teacher's desk was a large blackboard that stretched the complete length of the thirty-foot wall, equipped with chalk and erasers.

The teacher would draw lines dividing the chalkboard into four sections. He had to leave what he had written and use the next section for the next class because there weren't enough books for everyone in class. In front of the teacher's desk were four rows of desks. Each row represented a grade, just like the section on the blackboard. In the back of the room stood a potbelly stove. When the weather got cold, arrangements were made for one of the older kids to come in early and build a fire so the room would be warm by the time class started. If the room wasn't warm enough by the time class started, the teacher would have us move our desks in a circle around the potbelly stove. The teacher would read until we fell asleep. If the room wasn't warm enough after the first hour to teach class, we were sent home for the day. Most winters, we stayed home until spring.

We had four subjects we studied during the day—reading, writing, spelling and arithmetic. The older kids would also study history and English.

We did classwork until "recess." The school board would give us a fifteen-minute break at 10:00 a.m. for snack time. The only trouble was that most of us didn't have anything to snack on. We were never a group that wasted time, so naturally we played ball. Lunch was at noon and lasted until one. Each team was picked while we ate lunch. At 12:10 the game was on. At two o'clock we had another recess period of fifteen minutes. We played ball. At three o'clock, school ended for the day.

That was our daily routine Monday through Friday, except on Friday. When weather permitted we practiced softball from lunch until 3:00, when it was time to go home.

We all walked to and from school each day. On our way home you could smell and see smoke from the wood-burning cook stoves. The woman of each house would build a fire early in the day so the stove would be hot enough to cook on by suppertime. Supper would be ready between five and six o'clock every day. Our usual meal was "soup beans," cornbread, fried or cooked "taters" and a piece of hog meat.

The cook stove served two purposes in our home. The stove had four burners on top, a place to build a fire in the middle and an oven in the bottom. The stove also served as a hot water heater. On the left side of the stove was a space that held about two gallons of water. As the fire burned hot while cooking, the water on the left became very hot.

Our house was approximately twenty-four feet square; the front porch extended the full length of the house and wrapped around to the back door where a hand-dug well was built in for convenience.

Greasy Creek hollow was eight miles of dusty, dirt roads full of potholes from spring rains. There were three schools–upper, middle and lower Greasy. Each Friday, one of the schools would challenge the other to a softball game, provided someone in the neighborhood was off work that day and volunteered their time and truck to haul the players. Only the best players got to travel to the challenging school. All the other students got to go home.

When a challenging team came to our school, it was a social event. Everyone in the neighborhood showed up for the game—Grandpa and Grandma, Mom and Dad, brothers and sisters, aunts, uncles, newborn babies and all. It was a time set aside each month to visit old friends, make new ones, laugh and relax—precious moments in time for a coal mining community that had nothing to look forward to except hard labor with little pay.

Each Friday after school Mom would give me seventy-eight cents and send me to the country store just up the road. I would buy an eight-pack of sixteen ounce RC Cola for supper. Supper on Friday was like having a party. Chili, slaw, burgers, "taters" cut thin to make fries and an ice cold "pop" to wash it down with. Now you talk about good! If that wasn't enough, later on that night, just before dark, Mom would bake a cake from scratch with egg—beaten white icing. If I didn't know better, I would have thought we were rich.

During my sixth grade, progress had moved our community forward. The county was taking better care of our roads. At the mouth of Greasy, a big two lane concrete bridge replaced the old one-lane swinging bridge that stretched across the Big Sandy River.

Mountain land on Greasy was full of high quality coal. When the bridge was finished, coal companies began putting in "deep mines". Coal trucks were hauling coal before daylight and continuing into the night, six days a week. Roads were paved from Big Sandy Bridge to the fork at the head of Greasy.

Day after day, more people were moving to Greasy. At middle Greasy, construction began on a new school. During that summer we watched our two-room school taken down and destroyed.

At the beginning of my seventh grade, we were to begin riding the bus to our new school. I don't think my brothers, sisters and I looked forward to the new school. We simply accepted it because there was no other choice.

It was late August, first day of school. My life changed that day. I had entered a world of people that were full of hate—mean, cruel and dissatisfied because the cycle of life they were accustomed to had changed forever.

As long as no one interfered with the bus driver, you were allowed to do what you wanted on the bus. The bus driver's job was simple—transport students to and from school. There were bullies on the bus that would move from seat to seat aggravating everyone. The bus would arrive at school one-half hour before class started. That half-hour was like a living hell each day.

One morning during this thirty-minute period, we all were in our classroom because a light snow had fallen the night before. Two of the bullies spotted an old man with a cane making his way across the snow-covered playground to get to the store that was just above the school. They went after him and started kicking snow on him. One of the bullies kicked the old man's cane away, causing him to fall in the snow. They stood and laughed while the old man crawled over to his cane so he could get back up. The bullies threw snow and pulled at the man's clothes until he was off the playground. They returned to the classroom bragging to the others that they told the old man the school yard belonged to them and he was never to come that way again.

Our "old school" had two classrooms. The new school had eight different buildings. That was called "progress."

Teachers wouldn't show up until it was time to start class, because parents were unhappy with the change, and they would take their frustration out on the teachers before class if a teacher showed up early.

Being a teacher on Greasy was a very difficult task. Teachers were only paid to teach, but to keep their job they had to endure the problems they had with the parents. That could be more difficult than teaching the children.

As classes began each morning, the first thing our teacher would do was remove his paddle from the desk drawer and laid it on top of the desk where we all could see. The paddle was a one inch thick piece of wood about four inches wide and two feet long, with a carved hand grip on one side so he could swing the paddle with force. The paddle was there to intimidate us, but he was more than willing to use it if necessary. If the bullies destroyed the paddle before class started, that was not a problem. He could simply go out, cut a very flexible limb from a tree and lay that on top of his desk. There might have been three or four students in class that never felt that heartache, that suffering, that dissatisfaction our teacher released upon our "backside" for one reason or another. I was in high school when the state banished the paddle from schools.

I graduated eighth grade with a low grade of sixty percent, just enough to say that I passed.

Greasy Creek never changed that much in the last two years I was at school, but as a family we moved forward.

Our house was a small, two-bedroom house sitting on two acres of land. There was no indoor plumbing. During my year in eighth grade, Dad had gotten a better job with a larger coal company. How could one person's good fortune bring better days for so many?

Mom and Dad traded the old house for a cinder block home just above where the old school once stood. Our new home wasn't any bigger in size, but it had indoor plumbing and twenty-five acres.

It was late fall when we moved to our new home. We started moving on a Saturday morning. We had to finish by Sunday evening so Dad could take the truck back to work by Monday morning.

It was very exciting at first. By Sunday evening, rain had started to fall. No one could do anything right. Clothes were falling from the truck into the mud. We kept going. Just after dark we finished. Mom fixed us each a cup of hot cocoa. We sat around the table and talked and laughed about the struggle we had in our past, but the future ahead looked bright.

During our first summer, we started construction to double the size of our new home. We built a hog pen across the road and planted a garden at the lower side of the house. Life would bring my family many days of hard physical labor. My mother and father's future looked dark for so many years, but they knew that with the grace of God and hard work, they now could see the light of a new path of hope.

It was early fall of 1969. Squirrel hunting was a favorite pastime for most men. I always loved the mountain. I had received a shotgun the previous Christmas, so I was ready to join the hunt.

My grandpa, uncles and older brother always got together on Friday nights to prepare for the next morning's hunt. I always enjoyed listening to them. Grandpa's house sat in the main head of the left fork of Greasy. The closest neighbor lived one half of a mile back down the dirt road. The small house was snuggled in between the mountain, surrounded by large virgin timber. Up on the mountain, behind the house, the land was clear-cut for the family cemetery. As you came upon the back porch there was a shelf built along the wall with a mirror attached. Close to the back door was a hand-dug well. There was no indoor plumbing. When you went in for supper, you would go to the cook-stove in the kitchen, get the dishpan, dip out some hot water, go out on the back porch and wash and shave. If you needed to use the outhouse, it was about one hundred feet to the left of the porch, out in the woods. After everyone had finished washing, water was drawn from the well to refill the cook-stove.

The house had four rooms. Each room was about twelve feet square—kitchen, living room and two bedrooms. You could go through a trapdoor in the back bedroom down into the cellar, where Grandpa made room for an extra bed. After supper, we would go out on the front porch to relax and discuss life or to do a lot of bragging about the hunt that hadn't even taken place. Grandpa always said we killed more squirrels on Friday night than we ever did during the hunt.

The front porch was so small; there was only room for one chair. A large chair to the left would seat three. I would sit in the middle, with Grandpa on my right and Grandma on my left. My brother and uncle would sit on each corner of the porch in front of us.

As I close my eyes and travel through time back to a place that will live forever in my heart, I believe I can almost feel Grandpa sitting there beside me as he rolled a "Prince Albert cigarette"—laughing at my brother and uncle. The smell of smoke would bother me as he flicked the ashes from the cigarette, but it's a moment that will bring wonderful memories forever.

I can see Grandma sitting there with her shawl wrapped tight around her. There was a chill in the air from a light rain that had begun to fall. Fog was hovering down low in the trees and an owl was hollering in the distance. Daylight was slowly disappearing into the night.

An hour or so passed. I can still hear Grandma say, "Adam, you take your pocket knife with you in the morning."

"Why, Grandma?"

"So you can cut a peep hole in this fog. That way you can see a squirrel up in top of one of those big hickories."

Everyone started laughing. Then Grandpa said, "Let's go in and sit by the fire before we go to bed."

There were shadows dancing on the wall from a warm fire that lit up the living room. We all sat and watched the fire that burned so hot until it would soothe our minds to a state of relaxation, forgetting our worries of yesterday and thinking of only tomorrow.

I sat beside the fireplace on the floor where Grandma kept a large rock and a hammer for cracking hickory nuts. I would listen to each word that was spoken, hoping we would stay up all night watching the fire burn.

HIGH SCHOOL

Greasy had grown to probably two hundred families. The new school was a thing of the past.

Greasy Creek was located in Pike County. Pike County was a dry county. No alcoholic beverages were allowed, but Greasy had someone almost every mile that sold bootleg whiskey. Every place in the county was the same way.

For some reason it was always important for a drunk to be seen or heard for at least a half-mile radius of their home. It was like being ten-years old again, takin' a piece of candy that you were told not to, then making sure you ate it in front of your friends, because they knew it was wrong.

A few years later there was an election to see if the county should legalize the sale of alcohol. Everyone that didn't drink was scared that if it passed, the number of drunks would double. The law couldn't handle the problem now, so what would happen then? But the law was passed. It was now legal to sell alcohol in Pike County. Liquor stores went up along the entire main highway. Bootleggers were out of business within six months.

People who bought alcoholic beverages found that you could buy a case of beer at the grocery store. It must have taken the excitement out of buying alcohol, because more than half of the people quit drinking, and people who did drink spent more time in jail.

School never really meant much to me. The only reason I went was because Mom and Dad told me I had to. Almost everyone that lived there worked in a coal mine. I don't remember anyone, not even the teachers in high school, telling us that our education would make a difference in our future. I guess they thought if I didn't care why should they? Out of four and a half years of school, the only subject I got better than a C in was algebra. I knew how to do all the problems before the teacher had a chance to discuss the assignment. All other subjects I passed with C's or D's—most were D's.

I never understood English. I had to return to high school for an extra half year to pass English class before I could graduate. I finished my half-year of English and got my diploma in 1974.

LIVING IN NEW JERSEY

My brother lived in New Jersey. He called during March of that year and asked if I would like to visit him and his wife for a few months. The trout fishing was excellent in North Jersey. I didn't have anything to do and I was never one to pass up a fishing trip.

I got a job the first week of April and started work at G.R.M. Electronic. The job only paid minimum wage but I felt I was doing fine.

My brother had a little two-bed camper. Just after work on Friday, we would go up to the Pequest River in North Jersey and trout fish all weekend.

Richard had a 69 Plymouth Road Runner. He said if I had the transmission fixed, he would give me the car. After about a month, I had enough money. Now I had a car, and I decided to stay in New Jersey for a while. I found an apartment in Mount Holly, New Jersey, about six miles from where I worked.

I had a job, an apartment and a car. All I needed now was a girlfriend. Girls weren't difficult to find, but they were extremely hard to keep. During winter months, I seemed to have good luck keeping a girlfriend, but on the third Saturday in March, trout fishing season opened, and shortly after that my girlfriend would find someone new.

The first weekend of May 1975, Richard and I were planning a fishing trip to the Pequest River. Richard wasn't able to get off work until Saturday at noon. I told him that I would wash and wax the car, load the fishing gear, and pick him up so we could go fishing. I arrived back at the apartment around 10:30. My apartment was one of about twenty in one large building. I had to park in the back and walk around to the opposite side. My apartment was in the middle of the complex. It would take a few minutes for me to get my gear and even longer to walk out to the car and back. I loaded the car and went back to the apartment for a bite to eat. I was inside for about ten minutes.

I grabbed my jacket, for it was time to go fishing. As I entered the parking lot, I quickly realized my car was gone. I ran back into the apartment and called the police. They were in the parking lot within five minutes. I was sitting in the passenger seat of the patrol car when the officer put the information on the radio. In just a couple of minutes, a voice said, "We're chasing a white 69 Road Runner down the interstate. We're having trouble keeping up". A moment of silence, then a voice said, "We lost it".

I truly loved that car. A 69 Plymouth Road Runner with a 383-4 barrel carb, solid white, two black racing stripes on the hood, black interior, 4-speed, dual exhaust, and chrome wheels. That car was a true pleasure to put a shine on—even more exciting to drive. As I shifted the gears I could hear the roar of the exhaust, nothing but power that I controlled.

There was no insurance to collect. I was in a little trouble.

The next day I bought a 3-speed bicycle. Come Monday, I started for work a little earlier than usual.

A friend gave me a ride during bad weather, but for the next five months, that bicycle was my transportation. Richard told me of a young lady that had a Dodge Dart for $800.00 dollars and I bought it. It sure felt good to have four wheels for transportation instead of two. It was a little more expensive, but hey, winter was getting closer each day.

GOING HOME

Summer of 1976, Richard decided he had had enough of New Jersey, and he and his family were moving back home to Kentucky. I didn't really like New Jersey, so I packed my clothes and gave away what few things I had in the apartment. I was Kentucky bound.

Dad gave Richard land to put a house on, and I stayed in a building out back of Dad's house. The building had a bed, heater, and a sink. The outhouse was located about one hundred feet from the house in the woods.

I got a job at a motel in Pikeville as a desk clerk, a job that would last through the winter months. C&O Railroad was hiring laborers for track work. It was almost certain anyone that passed a physical had a job. I went down to the employment office and filled out an application. As soon as I was finished, they sent me to the doctor's office for a physical.

C&O Railroad called later that afternoon and told me to report to the railroad office at Shelbiana on Monday at 6:30 AM. I was walking on clouds, for I was about to make more money than I had every made.

In the spring of 1977, on Monday I reported for work at the railroad office as scheduled. After signing in, six other men and I loaded into a large king-cab work truck. The bed was filled with manual tools like five ton jacks, steel bars made for pulling spikes, forks for shoveling gravel, rail tongs for carrying steel, sledge hammers for driving railroad spikes, and a five gallon jug of drinking water.

Our destination for my first day's work was Johns Creek Mountain. C&O railroad simply cut a winding road that went up and around the side of the mountain until it reached the top. A sloping ridge went down the other side to the valley below.

We parked our truck on a dirt road close to the track and carried our tools for a thirty-minute hike up the mountain until we reached a damaged area. As we began to work, the sun was rising from behind the mountain. I always knew what physical labor was, or at least I thought I did, until now. By lunchtime, the steel bars were so hot I could feel the heat burning my hands through my work gloves. My clothes were wet with sweat, and my arms, legs, and back were hurting from bending over all morning.

We had thirty minutes for lunch. We found a shady spot under a tree, close to the track. Lunchtime gave us a chance to remove our hardhats. I was so exhausted I fell asleep before lunch was over. The men on the crew had a good laugh when they woke me to return to work. By the end of the day, I didn't think I would be able to get home. Every bone in my body was hurting. Quitting was not an option, for any man or woman that lived in the coalfields knew that hard labor was a way of life. So the next day I would rise for work again, only this time I would double the amount of food in my bucket.

By early winter, I was getting physically capable of working as long as anyone else who worked on the crew, or so I thought. One Friday afternoon about four o'clock, my crew received orders to join two other crews on John Creek Mountain to work a derail. Nobody on any crew wanted to hear those orders anytime, let alone on a Friday, because standing orders of the railroad stated that once you're ordered to work a derail, no one was allowed to leave the job site until the railroad was back in working condition.

My crew arrived on the mountain just before dark. As we got out of the truck, a wet snow began to fall. The foreman told us he had a portable buggy that fit the tracks for carrying tools. We hiked one half mile down the mountain to the jobsite. The other crew was already working. We grabbed our tools, removed our buggy from the track and joined the other men. A railroad man showed up about nine-o clock with a bag full of cold hamburgers. We didn't mind; we were starving. We took a few minutes for supper, and then returned to work, because there wasn't a dry spot on the mountain to sit down and take a break.

There were twenty men on the side of a mountain working by light of torches, not a dry piece of clothing among them. You could hear the chattering of teeth in between the pounding of sledgehammers as they drove spikes into the night. I lasted until about two in the morning, when I was physically unable to move my body. They stood me up against a pole close to where the men were working and put a torch in my hand. I must have fallen asleep standing there. About five in the morning, a man woke me taking the torch from my hand. He said we were finished and it was time to go home. That few moments of sleep gave me enough strength to get myself home where I would sleep for the next twelve hours.

Our job required us to work in all kinds of weather; if the temperature dropped to zero during the winter, or rose to one hundred in summer, we still had to work and work hard. There were only two ways of getting out of work. One was if the foreman said, "Grab your dinner bucket. I'll have a man drive you to your vehicle. It was nice working with you". The other was if you took off your hard hat that was issued when you started work, and handed it to the foreman. He would then politely tell a man to drive you to your vehicle.

It was Friday evening in the late summer of 1978. We were just finishing up a sixty-hour week when orders came to work a derail on Johns Creek Mountain. I weighed 185 pounds when I started working for the railroad, and I was down to 155. I knew I wasn't physically able to work another derail. That's when I handed my hardhat to the foreman.

FALLING IN LOVE

One Saturday in midsummer, about two months before I quit the railroad, I was going out for the evening. About three miles down Greasy; I turned left and went across the mountain and down Dry Fork. Approximately two miles down the road, I passed a home with a beautiful young lady sitting on the front porch with her father. I remembered her from high school. I turned around and drove back. I pulled into the parking lot. Angie had gone into the house. I knew her father only by name. I asked if it would be all right to ask Angie if she would like to see a movie with me that evening. He answered with a slight grin, "Why, yes." He called for Angie to join us on the porch. She must have heard our conversation, because when she came out, her face was flushed. Her smile captured my heart. I couldn't resist the excitement on her face, the feeling from her eyes. She stood about five feet two inches, one hundred and ten pounds, with short, curly, brown hair—a very beautiful woman. I asked if she would like to see a movie. She replied, "Allow me to change my clothes, and I'll be right with you".

We stopped on the way to the movies at McDonalds and got something to eat. The movie ended at nine, but the evening was young. I thought she was enjoying herself, so I asked if she would like to go dancing. That suggestion brought a smile to her face. She quickly agreed. We went to a small club in town. Neither of us liked to drink, but we did enjoy dancing. We danced until closing. Then I took her home and asked if she would like to go on a picnic the next day after church. With a smile, she replied, "Yes." Then I kissed her ever so lightly goodnight.

There were many more nights of dancing for Angie and I until the biggest dance of all. On November 23, 1978, we were married.

Angie's job transferred her to Paintsville, Kentucky just a couple of weeks after our wedding. The move wasn't bad because it was only an hour drive from Pikeville. I was without a job, so moving to Paintsville wasn't a problem. I took a job in a small factory just outside of town.

A few months passed, and we were blessed to hear the good news that Angie was expecting our first child.

By the late seventies the price of a ton of coal was increasing with each day. Pike County had high quality coal in her mountains. A coal rush was coming that would last until the late eighties. Strip mining was taking down the mountains. Anyone with a little money and the will to take a risk could start a coalmine with hopes of becoming rich, and a few did just that.

Rumors were spread that every fourth house in Pike County belonged to a millionaire. That was probably true, but in between each millionaire, there were clusters of trailers. Trailers were cheap and convenient. "Buy one today, move in tomorrow," was the dealership motto.

By early summer, my father gave us a piece of land. Angie and I purchased a used singlewide trailer and moved back to Greasy Creek. By that time, the population of Greasy had grown to around two thousand. People were moving to Pike County from all parts of the country to find their fortune in those beautiful hills that held Black Gold.

There was a small underground mining company close to our home. The company needed a night watchman, and I took the job while Angie stayed home and took care of herself and our unborn child.

During the summer, I had been looking for a better job. I finally found one with a large coal company with better pay and health insurance. Finding a job like this was heaven sent, especially at this time in our lives.

HEART DISEASE

I went for a physical, which was required by the company. I was waiting in the examining room as an elderly gentleman walked in. He went through the normal procedure of examinations. During the procedure, I was worried that he would find out about my hearing problem. After the exam, I could tell by his reaction that he had found out about my hearing problem. I just knew that I wasn't going to get that job. As the doctor slowly turned and looked me in the eye, he said, "Mr. Robinson, you have a bad heart." I knew this doctor didn't know what he was talking about. I was twenty-four years old, played tennis three times a week, rode a bicycle ten miles each weekend, and did grouse hunting in the Appalachian Mountains. (Ten miles was nothing to walk behind a good grouse dog.) But knowing all that, didn't stop that big lump from coming in my throat. The doctor continued to tell me that I had the worst heart condition that he had ever seen in a man my age, and that he couldn't recommend me for that job. By this time, that job was the last thing on my mind.

As I walked out of his office, the lump in my throat became very large. The lump, the fear, turned to tears by the time I reached my car.

I had to find out what exactly what was wrong with me. I had heard talk of a young doctor named Ronald Mann in Pikeville. His office was only a mile from where I was. By the time I reached his office, I had convinced myself that Doctor Jones didn't know what he was talking about. Doctor Mann entered the examining room where I was waiting. He was a young man in his thirties, standing about five and a half feet tall, with sandy brown hair, a full mustache, and a pleasant voice. I told him what Dr. Jones had told me and that I wanted a second opinion.

After listening to my heartbeat and two or three medical tests later, Dr. Mann was finished with his exam. By this time, I was feeling much better. I knew this young doctor straight out of medical school would find all this talk about a heart condition would be just a mistake on Dr. Jones' part.

Dr. Mann entered the room. I could tell by the smile on his face and the pleasant look that Dr. Jones was wrong.

As I sat quietly waiting for those words, I felt better. Dr. Mann said, "Mr. Robinson, my tests show that there is something wrong with your heart. I don't know what, but it's not that serious at this time. I would like to make an appointment with a heart specialist in Lexington, Kentucky." I agreed. His office made an appointment with Dr. Joseph Harkness at the Lexington Clinic.

One week later at 2:00 p.m., I was sitting in the waiting room of a doctor that was a heart specialist. I didn't want to accept the fact that there was something wrong with my heart. What would this do to my life? The door opened, and a tall, slender man in his forties with dark hair entered. He introduced himself as Dr. Harkness. He seemed to be a very pleasant man.

As we talked and went through the normal chitchat, he began to listen to my heartbeat. A few moments later, he turned and said, "Paul, your aortic value is stuck and it's not functioning properly. I'm going to have a few tests done, and then I can tell you more about your problem."

I thought to myself, if this man can tell me all of this just by listening to my heart, he is definitely the doctor I need. By this time, I had accepted that I was only 24 years old and had a heart condition.

Dr. Harkness returned after the tests were finished. He began to explain, "Paul, the aortic valve is stuck in the open position, which is letting blood build up in the heart. At this time your heart is very strong. It's keeping your blood flow at a normal rate." He said," Paul, we will sometime in the future have to correct this problem. We shouldn't have to do anything until your early forties. The longer we can put it off the better, Paul. I know your problem will not get any better, but technology will." He asked if I had any questions and told me to return annually for a checkup.

I left his office feeling that I would worry about my heart condition when I was forty. In reality, that's exactly what I did.

The year was 1979, in the fall my first child was born. We named her Brianna. I also got a job working for a large coal company in Eastern Kentucky.

Everything in my life was wonderful. My job was working out so well. In 1982, I was made foreman/boss on the tipple (processing plant). In that year, my son, Daniel, was born.

In 1984, I was still feeling great, working fifty to seventy hours a week, playing tennis three times a week, riding bikes, playing basketball on Sunday.

It was the first week of October of that same year; we stopped the tipple for lunch. All the other guys had left. I was doing a double check to make sure everything was secure. As I started to leave the tipple, a tremendous blow of pain hit my chest. It was like something had exploded inside my chest. I fell to my knees.

I couldn't speak. The sweat began to roll down my face. Then, almost as swiftly as the pain began, it stopped. Needless to say, I took the rest of the day off, went home and relaxed over the weekend. I went back to work on Monday, since the pain was only for five to ten seconds. By Monday, I had forgotten all about it.

Little did I know what was really happening to me. One week later, on Sunday, at 9:00 p.m., the family and I were sitting on the couch watching television. I wanted to use the bathroom before the movie started. I got up off the couch and went into the hallway, and there was a tremendous amount of pain in my chest. This was a steady, heavy pressure pain, not like it was before. I grabbed my chest and leaned up against the wall to rest, thinking it would go away. It continued into my left arm and down my left leg. I was standing in front of my bedroom. I eased my way onto the bed and lay down. Angie came in and said the movie had started, would I like to watch it? I told her I had a headache, would she bring me two Tylenol and a glass of cold water, thinking the Tylenol would help ease the pain. After about ten minutes, the pain slowly went away. After that battle, I was totally exhausted. I didn't remember anything until about 10:30 the next morning.

Angie came in and woke me. I asked her why she didn't get me up for work. She said, "I tried, you told me you weren't going in today." I got up to go out on the porch. When I started to walk, I couldn't move my left leg or my left arm very well. As we went out on the porch, Angie went to the mailbox near the road and got the mail. I had received a letter from Dr. Harkness stating that my last check up showed that my heart was getting larger and I needed to have a checkup every six months. I looked at Angie and told her it was time for the surgery now, and to please call Dr. Harkness and ask him to schedule it as soon as possible.

I was to check into the hospital on October 27, 1984. I arrived at two in the afternoon. They scheduled me for a heart cauterization the next day, to be performed by Dr. Harkness. After the procedure, Dr. Harkness came in and explained that my heart was getting too large and I was right to request surgery.

On November 1, 1984, a nurse came into my room and woke me. It was 6:00 a.m. She said it was time to take me down for surgery. I knew surgery was scheduled for 7:00 a.m. She asked if I would like something to make me sleep before I left the room. I said no, so they took me down to the prep room. They stripped me down and spread a thick green antibiotic over approximately thirty percent of my body. As I lay there and watched, I quietly asked the "good Lord" to give these folks all the help possible and to give me the willpower to face this surgery. As they were finishing inserting the last I.V. I felt a totally relaxing ease come to my mind. A nun from the hospital staff walked up beside me and said, "Don't worry; he's with all of us." After those words were spoken, I knew I didn't have anything to worry about. I was ready. A few minutes later, a gentleman positioned himself at the head of the table where I was lying. Nurses were getting into position on each side of me. They folded blankets and laid them on each side of my body, leaving my chest exposed. I could see a silver tray on wheels being pulled close to the table. Big lights were drawn down very close from overhead. Then I noticed a position at my right arm was open. As I was thinking those very thoughts, a gentleman in his late thirties was taking that position. He introduced himself as Dr. Donahue, the surgeon that I was told about a couple of days earlier.

As the surgical team chitchatted between each other about the upcoming presidential election, I was listening for every breath, watching every movement. Suddenly, Dr. Donahue looked at me and said, "Are you ready?"

I said, "Let's do it."

He looked to the lady on my left and said, "Scalpel." She handed him a small silver knife, straight across my chest. He looked at the gentleman that was standing at my head. These next three words are very vivid. "Put him under." As I looked up to see him, all I saw was a black rubber mask coming down, covering my mouth and nose. That was the very last thing I remember.

It must have been later in the day that they woke me. I could just make out that my family was standing beside the bed. I must have fallen back to sleep, because the next thing I remember was waking up again, curtains pulled around my bed, a block wall to my left and a TV on the wall. I could hear voices behind the curtain. I felt as if I had just awakened from a good afternoon nap. I could see the IV that was in me, but that was expected.

I was feeling good at this point. No pain, just total relaxation. I decided to watch TV. As the sound of the TV came on, the curtain came apart and Dr. Donahue walked in. He looked at me, then at the TV, then back at me. He smiled and left the room. I must have fallen asleep again because later two nurses woke me while trying to bathe me during the night. The lights were down low. There were no other sounds coming from behind the curtains. I must have fallen asleep again.

The next time I woke, the curtains were open. I was in a round room with all the beds facing the nurse's station in the center. Everyone in the room had these little blue boxes in their hand. I couldn't understand what they were until a nurse came over and told me it was time to start breathing exercises. She handed me a little blue box and instructed me to take a deep breath and blow into the box, which would help exercise my heart and lungs.

While I was awake I was doing breathing exercises, but for the most part I slept. On the third day, I was moved to the third floor in a private room. There my family (Mom and Dad) could stay with me during the day. I had asked my wife to go home and stay with our kids. The surgery was a success. The danger had passed. It was time for her to take my kids home. That way I would not worry about the children or her.

They brought me into the room. Mom and Dad were waiting for me. They told me Angie, Daniel and Bri had gotten home safely.

I wasn't talking much because any movement would totally exhaust me and I would fall asleep. I woke later that afternoon. Dad was sitting in a chair over next to the window. I could see him looking at me. I could tell he knew I was awake. He just sat there and looked at me. I wasn't able to talk, I think he knew any activity, even talking, was more than I could handle. About a half-hour had passed. Neither of us had said a word. The only way I could lay was flat on my back. I started to get serious pain between my shoulders. As I opened my eyes, Dad was pulling my pillow down under my shoulders. When he finished, he just stood there and looked at me. I said, "Thanks." He went over to his chair and sat down. I was really; really glad he was there. I was just as glad he wasn't trying to talk with me.

Another half-hour passed. Not a word was spoken. I fell back asleep. I often wonder about that evening. Dad, by nature, enjoys conversation. He sat there for an hour and a half—not a word. The movement of a pillow took pain from my back when I was unable to tell him what was wrong. I honestly believe the Lord was controlling his actions that evening.

Day four. When I woke, Mom and Dad were standing by the window. Dad turned and asked how I was feeling this morning. Would I like some breakfast? I said, "No."

Then Dr. Harkness walked through the door. He was smiling as usual. He said, "Good morning, Paul. Hope you are feeling okay."

As I said, "I'm a little sore," he said good morning to Mom and Dad. Then he began to examine me. After he finished he said, "Paul, your recovery has been excellent. I was talking with Dr. Donahue. He said the surgery was a complete success. Paul, your heart is in very good condition. You should live a very long life. Now, what I want you to do is to get up and start walking. Call a nurse, or your Mom and Dad can help you, but we need to start exercising that heart muscle and keep those lungs cleaned out."

As he left the room, I decided to start right away. I was tired of lying in that bed and not being able to move. I simply wanted to go to the bathroom without help. I started to get up. Mom and Dad helped me out of bed. I was finding it difficult, not because of the pain (medication was taking care of that), mostly because I was so weak. I made it to the bathroom and back "okay", but it left me totally exhausted. When I lay back down, I could hear the valve inside my heart. I could hear it before. It was just a weak noise. I didn't pay much attention until now. It sounded like the old windup alarm clock at Grandma's house that went tick-tock during the night. Only now, that clock was in high speed and twice as loud. Knowing there was a mechanical valve inside my heart making that noise, yet it was still my heart, was a strange feeling. It was quiet. The only thing I could hear was the sound of my heartbeat. The sound became very aggravating. In my mind, I knew that the sound would be a constant reminder of what had taken place with me. The heart is an extremely vital organ that exists inside all of us. One that "God" had placed so carefully in the center of our chest, wrapped in a mass of bones that shield and protect. Mine was no longer perfect. I knew that my heart wasn't perfect before the operation, but now I knew it would remind me every day.

Later in the afternoon, I woke and saw Mom and Dad sitting in the chairs next to the window. We talked for a few minutes, and then I asked them to go home. The nurse would help me walk. I was doing much better and didn't need anyone to stay with me. They packed their things, said they would call when they got home, and left. Not long after they left, Dr. Donahue came in. We didn't talk much. He examined me and told me my heart sounded great.

Day five, the nurses were coming in on a regular basis to check on me, and to help me in and out of bed so I could go to the bathroom or simply to turn me over. I knew what I had been through, but I didn't expect such VIP treatment. One would think that I was a king or president instead of a simple coal miner from Eastern Kentucky.

Later on in the afternoon, I had a visitor. Angie had a sister that lived in the neighborhood. I had only met her for a brief moment before, but I did recognize her when she walked in. I felt as if I should be a good host for my visitor. The nurses had helped me get cleaned up. I was presentable, but I felt very dirty because I had lain in bed for so long. Gay, Angie's sister, only stayed for approximately five minutes. It felt like an hour. I had been in the hospital for seven days. Please believe me when I tell you those were the worst five minutes I had while being there.

Day six, I'm awake when they brought in breakfast. I had eaten very little, if any, until now. This morning I was getting hungry. I wasn't able to eat what they had brought. When the nurse came in, I asked if she would order me a couple of big oranges. She left the room, and about three minutes later, a man from the cafeteria brought the oranges. They were delicious. From that day to the end of my stay in the hospital; I ate oranges for breakfast, lunch and supper.

It wasn't long after breakfast when Dr. Harkness came in. I had been visiting Dr. Harkness about eight years now. He always had a smile and was in a good mood. Today wasn't any different. A doctor in his position that takes care of people twenty-four hours a day, seven days a week, has more problems to solve than any three average people do. But when he would come in to check on me, I would feel there were no others patients. His only concern was my well being. "Today I'm starting you on coumadin," he said. "It's a type of medicine that helps prevent blood clots from forming on your valve inside your heart. If you should get cut, it would take twice as long for the bleeding to stop than it would have before the operation. Your blood will clot. It will just take longer. Pro-time count in a person averages around twelve. With this medication, I'm raising yours to the average of twenty to twenty-four, on your pro-time count. When you leave the hospital, go to your family doctor. Get your blood checked once a month, making sure it averages twenty to twenty-four on your pro-time count. If it doesn't, your doctor should increase or decrease your medication. Never ride a motorcycle or use a chainsaw." I think he explained to me about ten times how important it was for me to take my medication and get my blood checked each month.

Medication, getting my blood checked every month-I guess that wasn't too bad for what I had been through. I asked if there was anything more that would interfere with my heart. Dr. Harkness said, "Paul, you should live a normal life and grow old successfully with this valve".

I didn't have any doubts about the operation. Nor did I have any doubt about a full recovery. After Dr. Harkness left the room, I got out of bed, went to the bathroom and washed my face, and then went for a walk.

Day 13, I was getting strong by now, staying awake for most of the day, walking a lot, getting on everyone's nerves. I wanted to go home. Dr. Harkness came in the first thing that morning. I asked how much longer I would have to stay in the hospital. Dr. Harkness said, "Paul, I would have let you go home sooner if you lived near the hospital. Since you live three and a half hours away, you had to stay longer. As of now, your coumadin level is where it needs to be so you can go home tomorrow."

Those were the words I wanted to hear. He finished examining me and left the room. I picked up the phone, called Angie, and told her to send someone for me tomorrow. I was getting out of the hospital first thing in the morning.

The days weren't very long until now. I was excited. I stayed awake the whole day. The next morning, I was up and ready before breakfast. Dr. Harkness came in and told me about my medication again and that I was to return in about three months to his office at the clinic.

My brothers arrived shortly after. We left the hospital about eleven o'clock and arrived home about three in the afternoon. Angie prepared the bed. She had to wait until I got home because I brought a foam mattress home that the hospital gave to me. After about thirty minutes, I fell asleep. I didn't wake up until the next day.

BACK TO WORK

For the first couple of days, I walked through the house. After that, I started walking outside. At first, I could only walk one tenth of a mile, then go back in and rest for about three hours. On my fifth day, I walked about a half mile up the road. On my second week, I was walking two miles a day. On my fourth week, I was getting restless. I had too much energy. The company I worked for called and invited me to the company Christmas party. I told Angie that I was going back to work. I would prove to the company that I was ready for work.

We attended the party on Friday night. Angie liked to dance, so it wasn't hard to get her on the dance floor. We arrived at eight o'clock, danced five or six times, socialized a lot, and left the party at midnight. Physically, I felt great, but I was ready for bed. I knew I had succeeded by the look on everyone's face.

Sunday afternoon the phone rang. It was the president of the company. They were holding a meeting this evening. Would I attend?

The company had bought a new tipple in West Virginia on the Kanawha River. I was to report Monday morning at nine o'clock. It was exactly six weeks after my open-heart surgery. For the first week, I was to open the gates and let coal trucks bring in coal and stockpile for loading barges on the river. I reported back in Kentucky on Friday with a record showing how much coal was stockpiled and ready for shipping.

The company decided to send a complete crew on Monday to load barges for shipment. My official job was to be on the river to load the barges properly. The weather had turned cold. Wind blowing off the river turned temperatures to about zero degrees. After the shift was over, we headed back to the motel for showers. Then we all went to supper.

After supper, everyone was sitting around talking. I decided to go back to the room and turn in early. I was sharing a double with a co-worker. I checked with Bobby (the co-worker) to make sure he had a key. He always sat around and had a beer before he turned in.

I arrived at the hotel, turned on the TV and got ready for bed. I took the top blanket and folded it where I could lay on it because the mattress was too hard. I took two pillows and laid them long ways where they would go under my shoulders for extra softness. I lay there for about thirty minutes watching TV when all at once a very hard pain came between my shoulder blades and went through into my chest. It was like the inside of my chest was in a perfectly round vice that was closing very slowly. The pressure was so extreme I was having trouble breathing. I was turning side to side, trying to relieve the pressure. I couldn't move my arms enough to reach the nightstand where my pain pills were. All at once the door opened. Bobby walked in and asked what was wrong. As I pointed to the pain pills on the nightstand, he knew I was in trouble.

Bobby helped me take a pain pill. Within thirty seconds, the pain was completely gone. I fell asleep and didn't wake up until the wake-up call came the next morning. Everything went okay the rest of the week. We returned home for the weekend. I didn't tell my family about what happened, because it wasn't necessary for them to worry.

Saturday night, about two o'clock in the morning I started to cough. Each time I coughed the pressure would pull on my chest. The cough continued for about twenty minutes. I couldn't handle the pain any longer. It felt like the bones in my chest were coming apart each time I coughed. Angie called Dr. Mann, my family doctor. He suggested one tablespoon of whiskey. I don't drink, but a co-worker had gotten me a bottle of whiskey a couple of years earlier. As soon as I drank that whiskey, the cough went away. Man, you should have heard me thanking that guy for that present.

I continued working in West Virginia for two more months. Everything went fine. I didn't have anymore-serious pain. It was early March. I had to report back to work in Kentucky. That was fine by me. I didn't like working on that river. I was happy to be back home.

FIRST CHECKUP AFTER SURGERY

I had an appointment with Dr. Harkness at the end of the month. Fear was what I felt on the first day that I learned I had a heart condition. After that, I knew everything would be okay. Knowing it was time for my first check up after the surgery was the second time I felt afraid of what might happen. I didn't want to go back into the hospital, surgery, more tests, nothing, and nothing. All I wanted was for this to go away. I wanted my life back to normal. Basically, it wasn't until I started thinking about going back to the doctor's office that everything I went through came back to haunt me. In my mind, I thought that the same thing could happen all over again. I didn't tell anyone what I was thinking at that time, but I was very difficult to live with for the month of March.

My appointment was at eleven o'clock. I liked to make all of my doctor appointments as early as possible. That way, once I get up to start my day, I would consider it a job. That's what I had done from day one.

I had a three and a half hour ride ahead of me. Angie drove me down. As I entered the waiting room, I started to relax a little. I began to realize it was just another visit to the doctor. I hadn't had any serious pain for a while. I felt good.

The nurse called me back to the exam room. Shortly after, Dr. Harness came in. We started to talk. He did his exam. As I was putting my shirt on, he said, "Paul, you have made a remarkable recovery. Your heart sounds great. I'll make another appointment for you in six months."

That day was a great day for me. I had fought the biggest battle of my life. I went through the surgery, went back to work, and three months later, the checkup was, in my mind, the last battle. I had won.

MOVING TO VIRGINIA

For the first year after surgery, I had some pain. It was expected–not enough to think about twice. I would only talk about the operation when someone would ask me a direct question. Work had started to slow down. To make ends meet, I started building porch swings.

A couple of years passed. The mine where I worked shut down because of lack of business. My company wasn't the only one. Things got bad. A newspaper advertised that a mining company was taking application for thirty-two positions. The news on the radio reported later that 3,000 miners showed up for those jobs.

The year was 1989. I had been out of work for about two years. Our only income was Angie's job. She was working, but her rate of pay was minimum wage, $4.25 per hour. Things were looking bad. I called the unemployment office in Radford, Virginia. They told me the unemployment rate was three percent. There were plenty of jobs there.

I left Kentucky on Wednesday. On Thursday, I went to work as a construction worker. I stayed with friends while I worked. I went home on weekends. After about a month, I got a better job working in a factory. Shortly after that, Angie and the children joined me. We rented a house in Pearisburg, Virginia. Angie had only been here for a few days, and she went to work. It wasn't easy, but it was looking better. The house we rented had a full basement. I decided to continue building furniture. By this time, I had designed a complete deck set—chairs, loveseat, picnic table, coffee table and gliders to match.

A year passed. Angie and I had gotten enough money together for a down payment on a house. We were working. We had bought a used doublewide trailer with almost two acres of land. The kids were happy in their new school. Everything looked good.

BLESSED

I decided to start a small business designing and building my furniture on a part-time basis. I started my business in the spring of 1991. I would work, building my furniture in the morning and working at the factory in the evening. I had been doing this for about two months, when one evening while at the factory, I got a very serious pain in my left shoulder and arm. My whole body was sweating. The pain only lasted for about thirty seconds. I decided to get the boss to have someone run me over to the hospital and have him or her check me over. I went through a series of tests, but they came up empty. All tests came back normal.

About one month later, while working building furniture, I felt a little weak. That wasn't unusual, but what happened next was. I had completely lost my voice. If there were five words in a sentence, I could feel myself speaking the words, but only the last word in the sentence was vocal. I couldn't understand why I couldn't speak. I felt okay. I didn't have any pain. I felt completely normal. I just couldn't speak.

My sister and her husband (Joyce and Roy) came up for a visit. It was on a Saturday. They came by the shop to talk for a while. Only I couldn't speak. They didn't understand. If nothing was wrong with me, why wasn't I able to speak? I would write down everything. After awhile, they began to laugh when I would try to speak. Even I began to laugh about it, mostly because I didn't understand what was happening to me. About three hours had passed from the time I lost my voice, my sister suggested that I should go home and get some sleep. We left and went home. I just pointed to the bedroom, went in and lay down. Later in the evening, when I woke up, my voice was back to normal.

I called Dr. Harkness' office on Monday and explained what had happened with my voice. They put me on hold. A few minutes later a voice said, "Paul, this is Dr. Harkness. Please come down first thing Tuesday morning and report to the emergency room at Saint Joseph Hospital. I will be waiting for you there."

I went down to Kentucky and stayed overnight. Mom and Dad drove down to Lexington with me the next morning. We arrived at approximately at the emergency room at 10:30 a.m. I gave my name and insurance card at the front desk.

The lady said they had been waiting for me. I didn't think it was such a big deal. I felt great.

About sixty seconds passed. I didn't even have time to sit down in the waiting room when two nurses came from behind the swinging doors pushing a "bed". They instructed me to lie down. Within minutes, I was in an examining room with wire and machines hooked all over my chest. Within another sixty seconds, Dr. Harkness walked in and started asking questions while he examined me. I told him that the only problem I had was that I lost my voice for about five hours on Saturday, but everything else was fine. No pain, nothing. After I took a nap, I was back to normal. He explained to me that when someone has a stroke, they lose the ability to speak. Four hours later, a series of test concluded that I had had a light stroke.

Dr. Harkness told me that my "pro-time" was low. There was a blood clot trying to form on the heart valve. Sometime during the beating of the heart, the clot broke loose from the valve and lodged somewhere else, causing me to lose my voice. After a while, the clot deteriorated. There was no permanent damage done, but that's what caused me to lose my voice.

I returned home and went back to work the next day. I also went back to the family doctor to get my blood "PT" checked. He increased my medication.

It was mid-July that year on a Saturday, just after lunch. I was working on a picnic table at my shop, about thirty minutes from my home. The weather was hot. I was bending over to tighten a bolt, when I felt something move in my chest. It moved very quickly for about four inches. Then it stopped. As it moved, it was hurting, but when it stopped, the real pain started. It was like someone had taken away the air I was breathing. I was gasping, but I couldn't find the oxygen. At the same time, it felt as if there were a thousand pounds lying on my chest. I was lying on the floor with my back against the picnic table. As the pressure was building, the pain was severe. I don't understand what happened next. I couldn't feel the pain any longer. I could see my body lying there. I didn't have the air to breathe. I could see my body, but I couldn't feel it at all.

I think when the Lord made the human body; he gave our brain the capability of blocking out pain that our mind can't endure. Only a few moments later, the pain came back into my chest. By this time, I was getting some air to breathe. I could feel the pain starting to relax in my chest. A few moments later, the pain was gone. I was back to breathing normally, but I was exhausted. I couldn't move. I must have fallen asleep.

Later that afternoon, I awoke lying beside that picnic table on a concrete floor. I got up and walked around for a while. I got a Pepsi to drink. After I was finished with my drink, I felt as if nothing had ever happened, so I just went back to work.

In the spring of 1992, I quit my job at the factory and started working full time building my furniture. I was working ten hours a day, seven days a week, stocking up for spring.

It was around eight o'clock one evening. I had come home, taken a shower, and I was relaxing on the couch. Brianna came over and sat beside me. As she sat there with her head on my chest, it occurred to me that I hadn't realized how fast she was growing. She was twelve years old and would become a teenager the following summer. Then it would be only a short period of time until she was ready for college.

About that time she raised her head, looked at me and said, "Daddy, I can't hear the beat." I hadn't heard my heartbeat for some time. Then I fell asleep.

The next morning when I woke, I felt just fine and needed to get to work. I never thought about that evening again.

At the beginning of March, I slowed down on my work, because I was getting migraine headaches about once a week. When I got a migraine, I would get an upset stomach, sometimes even to the point where I would throw up or have a fever. My head would hurt so badly that I couldn't move it from one side to the other without creating an enormous amount of pain. My eyes would become very sensitive to light. The only way I could help myself was to find a very cool and dark room with absolutely no noise, take two Tylenol and go to sleep for a couple of hours. After I would wake, the headache would be gone, but the soreness in my head would last two or three more hours.

About the beginning of April, Mom and Dad came up for a visit. They stayed for a few days. It was Saturday. They decided to go home. When they left, I decided to go to work. It was a short time after I arrived at work that Dad came walking through the door, and I asked if something was wrong. He told me that they had driven about five miles toward home when something told him he needed to go back. "So we came back to your house. Everything was okay there, so I decided to come up here to your shop and check on you."

I was tired and I told him to wait for a few minutes until I locked up, because I wasn't feeling well. I would ride home with him and pick my truck up later.

By the time we started home, I had lost my voice again. I could only speak about one word in ten. By the time we arrived home, I was feeling okay, but I couldn't speak. Dad tried to get me to go and see a doctor, but I refused. I went in the bedroom and lay down to take a nap. When I woke, I was back to normal.

I was working well, but the headaches were about twice a week now. I got a little, fold-up bed to put in the back room of my shop so I could stay there when they occurred. One day in the afternoon, about the last of April, I was at work when the phone rang. It was my brother calling from Kentucky. He was planning a fishing trip. He called to ask if I would like to go. We were on the phone for about ten minutes when all at once, the room started to turn. My head was spinning so fast it gave me an upset stomach. I told my brother that my stomach was upset and I needed to hang up and go get something to drink. After I drank a glass of water, I was okay so I went back to work.

It was about the first week in May. I was loading the truck with furniture for a delivery when I got really dizzy and had to sit down for a few minutes. I got a drink of water and everything was back too normal.

By the middle of May, my headaches had increased to about one every other day. I was working a lot of hours at this time. Memorial Day weekend was about three days away, and I needed to get a lot of furniture ready, but I was having a problem. I couldn't walk fifty feet without sitting down. I thought I was working too hard. I decided that I would work through the weekend, then take a couple of days and catch up on my sleep. I made it just fine until Saturday. I had a delivery to make first thing that morning. When I arrived at the shop, I started to load the truck. Just as I finished, I got short of breath and very dizzy. I had to sit down for a few minutes. Then I got a drink of water and was up and ready to go again.

My delivery was only about three miles from my shop. When I arrived, a man and his wife in there sixties were mowing the lawn. They stopped to help me unload the furniture. We each got a chair to carry. We had to walk down a hill about fifty yards, go around the lower side of the house, then up a stairway of about twenty steps to their deck. I made it about halfway, and then I had to sit down and rest. After about five minutes I made it up to the deck. By the time I reached the top, I had very little air to breathe, and I was so dizzy I was leaning up against the wall. I slid down to the floor. I couldn't see anything. Everything was like a deep foggy rain in the mountains, except all the fog was in my mind. I sat there a few minutes until I was feeling better. The gentleman asked if I would like to come in and get something to drink and he would pay me.

After I arrived back at work I decided to call a doctor. I didn't want just any doctor. I felt I needed a heart specialist. I called one hospital that was very large in size, but they didn't have a heart specialist. I asked if they knew a hospital nearby that would have a heart specialist. They recommended Radford Hospital; about thirty minutes drive from my shop. I called and asked to speak to a heart specialist. A man came on the phone and introduced himself as Dr. Wyne. He asked if he could help. I told him about my operation. Then I told him what was happening to me at the present time. He asked when would I like the appointment. I said "Right now." He told me to come to the emergency room. He would be waiting for me there.

I left my shop and drove straight to the hospital. I had to park in the hospital parking lot, which was about three hundred feet from the emergency room. I decided to walk very slowly so I wouldn't get dizzy. I could make out a chair to my left as I entered the hospital. I sat down there. After a few minutes, everything became clear and back too normal. I introduced myself to the receptionist at the front desk and told her Dr. Wyne told me to report to the emergency room. She said, "Mr. Robinson, we've been expecting you. Please go through the door on your right."

I walked into the room. A young lady said, "Mr. Robinson, please have a seat." The room was very small-just a hallway in front of me. To my left was a miniature nurse's station with two seats. As I sat down, the nurse began to call Dr. Wyne to inform him of my arrival. She began to get the necessary information for the hospital records. After that, she began to take my vital signs. Then she asked, "Mr. Robinson, how did you get here today?" I told her that I had driven my truck. She informed me that was very dangerous, that my pulse was only thirty-nine and my blood pressure was extremely low.

"Mr. Robinson, Please come with me. I'll take you to an examining room where Dr. Wyne will meet with you."

As we left her station, we went into a big hallway with rooms on each side. We took the first door to the right. As we entered the room, a nurse was working with a machine. She turned and introduced herself, as the other nurse left the room. She asked if I would please lie down on the bed that was in front of me. As I lay down, she explained to me that Dr. Wyne told her to do an echocardiogram and an EKG.

As she was hooking up the machines, the door opened. A middle-aged man walked in. He stood about 5'6" and was very slim. He had on a long white jacket. As he introduced himself, he was speaking very loudly, which was great because I couldn't hear very well anyway.

"Mr. Robinson, my name is Dr. Wyne. We spoke on the phone. As I look at your chart, you stand at 5'9" tall and you weight 176 pounds. From looking at you, you look like you are in very good shape, but you tell me that you can't walk any distance at all without getting dizzy or short of breath."

"That's correct, Doc," I said.

Then he turned to discuss the readout of the test with the nurse. I lay there in silence, waiting, hoping and listening for any words of encouragement. Dr. Wyne turned and went out the door. Only moments later, he returned. Two other gentlemen came in behind him. The two gentlemen, Dr. Wyne, and the nurse discussed the readout of the echocardiogram. I watched and waited. Only minutes had passed. The two gentlemen turned and left the room. Dr. Wyne looked at me. "Mr. Robinson, we have found your problem. You have a blood clot inside your heart. This clot is cutting off the flow of blood to the rest of your body. That's why you're having dizziness and shortness of breath."

"Mr. Robinson, the only way we know of removing that clot in your heart is by open heart surgery."

By nature, I smile a lot. When I meet people I smile. They seem to feel more relaxed about talking with me. So I have a habit of smiling.

When Dr. Wyne told me about needing surgery, he was somewhat confused and asked, "Mr. Robinson, how can you sit there and smile when I'm telling you that you're going to have to have surgery again?"

I told him that surgery was not going to happen. I don't know why I'm saying this, but surgery will never happen. I knew by his reaction when he continued to talk, that I was in denial about surgery. Even at that moment, I knew that surgery was not even a possibility. I was not upset, aggravated or even disturbed by this problem.

Dr. Wyne continued to explain to me about a Roanoke hospital that specialized in "open heart" surgery. I requested that I be sent back to Lexington, Kentucky, where Dr. Harkness practiced.

Dr. Wyne couldn't understand why I would request to be sent back to St. Joseph Hospital, which is a six hour trip, when I could travel forty-five minutes to a hospital that does "open heart" surgery.

Dr. Wyne continued to explain. With the clot in my heart, he couldn't allow me to leave the hospital. I was in critical condition. If I insisted on going back to Kentucky, I would be transported by ambulance, but for now he was admitting me until the arrangements could be made. I agreed.

I was transported down the hall to a private room. A nurse came in and took a blood sample. I was hooked to one machine that was monitoring my heart. Only moments later, another nurse was starting an IV. When that was done, I called Angie and told her where I was and what was happening.

About thirty minutes had passed. Dr. Wyne returned to my room. He began to explain that he had made several phone calls. "First, I have called St. Jude. They explained to me everything about your heart valve. Second, I have spoken with Dr. Harkness in Lexington and told him of your problem. I have started you on a blood thinner through the IV that takes effect immediately, so your heart can work easier with that clot. I explained to Dr. Harkness that your pro-time is extremely low and I've already started you on this medication. I've also told him of your request to be transferred to St. Joseph Hospital. He told me to call him with a scheduled time of arrival. He would be there waiting for you. I cannot allow you to be taken off the medication. You will need to be transferred by ambulance. I checked. You do have insurance through your wife's work I will sign, saying that this is a critical matter. I'm not trying to cause you any financial problems. This has to be done to protect your life. I've explained this to Dr. Harkness and he has agreed with me."

Dr. Wyne asked if I had any questions. I asked, "When will I be transferred to St. Joseph". He said he would schedule it as soon as he finished talking to me.

Then he asked, "How long has it been since you took your medication?"

I explained that it had been about eight days. He asked why I had stopped taking the medicine. I said I had a lot of different reasons, but mostly it was just stupidity on my part.

Dr. Wyne explained that it would have taken longer those eight days to form a clot that size in my heart.

Then he said, "I'll see you in a couple of hours," and left the room.

The afternoon passed slowly. I had a few friends stop by. Angie, Daniel and Bri came over and stayed the afternoon with me. Dr. Wyne came in and told me that he had scheduled my transfer to St. Joseph for nine o'clock Sunday morning.

Angie wanted to go to Lexington on Sunday, so she asked friends to come over to the house and take care of Daniel and Bri until she returned.

Everyone had left by six o'clock so I watched television until about ten. Then I fell asleep. I slept through the night. The next morning I was awake by the time breakfast was served. I was up and ready to go. Waiting is not one of my strong points. Angie came in shortly after Dr. Wyne entered the room. He told me that the ambulance would be here shortly. They would be able to monitor my heart and continue the medicine. Dr. Wyne wished me good luck and then left the room. Friends came in to visit. We sat and talked. About thirty minutes later, the ambulance crew showed up. Angie was driving her car down shortly after that. We were on our way.

The ambulance ride was interesting at first, but after the first thirty minutes, it was starting to get boring. The rain had begun to fall in very heavy downpours at times. We had to travel through Beckley and Charleston, West Virginia. Mountain area fog would be so heavy on some of the mountains that visibility would only be twenty or thirty feet.

Needless to say, I was sitting up by this time. A thousand things were going through my head. "Had I made the right choice? Angie is somewhere behind us. Her eyesight is not very good. This weather isn't helping. I already caused her too much heartache with my condition. She should not have to suffer because of me. I guess love is kind of like this fog; it is so overwhelming and beautiful and totally out of our control. Well, this will be a long trip if I don't do something besides sit here and make mountains out of molehills with every thought. Maybe they will let me drive this ambulance. I think I'll ask. If nothing else, it will break the ice for some conversation."

We arrived at St. Joseph Hospital about three in the afternoon. As the ambulance attendants pushed me through the door, to my surprise there stood my father, my mother, my sister and her husband. I think they felt a lot better about me when I sat up to talked with them. They explained that Angie had called them yesterday and told them of my condition. As we talked, two nurses came over. They changed me from the ambulance bed to the hospital gurney. Then a nurse said, "Mr. Robinson, we have a room for you on the third floor. Dr. Harkness will be there by the time we get you up there."

We entered the room. They had me into bed within seconds. They took off the machine that the ambulance had hooked up and hooked up two others. I could see my family standing at the door while the nurses worked. Only moments had passed when Dr. Harkness came in. We chitchatted, while the nurses were running tests. He turned to check the test results, and then looked back at me.

"Paul, you definitely have a blood clot inside your heart. We will need to operate to remove the clot as soon as possible."

I told Dr. Harkness that I didn't want another operation; there should be some other way. Dr. Harkness told me to think about it. He would be back within the hour.

The nurses finished their work. One stopped to explain that I was being monitored from inside the nurse's station. "Someone will be in to check on you about every ten to fifteen minutes."

As the nurses left the room, Mom and Dad, with my sister and her husband, entered the room. I was still sitting up. We talked for a while. Then Angie walked in. That lifted a lot of pressure from my mind. We talked for about twenty minutes. Then Dr. Harkness came in. He asked the family to leave the room so he could talk with me alone.

Dr. Harkness began to explain, "Paul, we have medication that we could give you. It takes three hours to administer through your IV. This drug will go on and bust up the blood clot into very small pieces and hopefully dislodge it. You have about the same chance of this working as you would with surgery."

I didn't have a second thought. I answered immediately. "Give me the medicine."

In my mind and in my heart, I knew that this was what I was looking for. I knew that the medication would work the very minute Dr. Harkness told me about it. He told me that they would start the medication about seven o'clock. I told him that was fine with me. After he left, the family came in. I told them what was planned.

We talked for a while. Then Mom and Dad decided to go next door to get a hotel room for the night. My sister and her husband did the same. Angie decided to stay with me in the private room that I was in.

Around five o'clock, the nurses' shift had changed. A nurse walked in and introduced herself. She informed me that she would be taking care of me for the next eight hours. I enjoyed the way she talked.

Then I asked, "Are you from down under?"

"I am Australian," she replied. We talked for a few minutes and then she left the room. Angie was sitting in a chair next to my bed almost asleep, tired from the drive down.

The lady from down under came in about every ten minutes to check on me. I must have fallen asleep, or else time passed very quickly, for the next time *Australia* came in, she said, "I'm starting the medicine that Dr. Harkness told you about. If you need anything, please push the 'nurse' button," then she left the room. Time passed. I don't know how long, but Australia was in and out of my room asking how I was feeling. I told her that I was getting a steady pain in my left side toward my back. I asked for a couple of Tylenol for the pain.

After a few minutes, she was back with the Tylenol. Some time had passed. The pain in my side was getting worse. I tried to watch some television, but it didn't help. The TV was changing programs. It must have been eight o'clock. The pain was a heavy, steady pressure now. *Australia* walked back in. I asked if I could have something stronger for the pain. She replied that it would take a couple of minutes to talk with Dr. Harkness. About five minutes passed. *Australia* walked in with a couple of tablets. I didn't ask what they were, I just took them, hoping the pain would go away. I watched TV for about twenty minutes, trying to give those tablets time to work. By this time, I was turning from side to side. No matter what position I would put my body in, the pain was only getting worse. I couldn't lay still. I asked *Australia* if I could take something else for the pain in my side. By this time, she was almost staying in the room with me. She said, "I'll call Dr. Harkness. Give me a couple of minutes." She came back in with a syringe about half full of medication. I tried to give the medicine time to work, but I couldn't handle the pain. I was starting to scream with pain. There were moments of relief. As *Australia* walked in, I told her that I couldn't handle the pain. "Please call Dr. Harkness. Get me some help."

A few minutes later, she returned with another syringe almost full. As she gave me the shot, she said a few words and started to walk away. I could barely see her as she left the room.

I woke up about three hours later. The pain was gone. I felt much better. Exhausted from the battle, I thought to myself, "The good Lord has let me win another one," for I could hear the valve in my heart click like the clock on the wall. A few moments had passed. Then *Australia* walked in and asked how I was feeling. I told her that my side was very sore, but I felt good. The medicine must have worked.

Australia left the room. I fell back to sleep. The next morning, someone that brought in breakfast awakened me. Angie was reading a book in the chair next to my bed. I sat up, had breakfast and talked with Angie for about twenty minutes. Then Dr. Harkness came in. "Paul, the nurse told me that you could hear your heart valve." Then he smiled. "I'd like to listen, then I'll have the nurse come in and do another echocardiogram. If any of that clot is left in your heart, a little more medicine should take care of it, but your heart sounds good. We'll know more after the test."

After Dr. Harkness left the room, a young nurse came in, pulling a very large machine behind her. She introduced herself and told me that she was there to do the echocardiogram. We talked while she hooked me up to the machine. We chitchatted while she ran the test. As she was finishing up, I asked if the test showed any clot in my heart. As she turned her machine off, she looked at me and said, "Mr. Robinson, Dr. Harkness will read this report and let you know the results. We're not allowed to discuss any tests with any patients."

I couldn't control myself, so I asked again, "Do you think the test looks good?" She winked and smiled, then left the room.

After that, I had no doubt that the medication was a total success. I was weak, but my sprits were high. Angie and I talked for a while. Then another nurse came in, introduced herself and asked if I needed anything. I explained to her that the medicine that I was taking for the soreness in my side was making me sleep too much. I asked if I could get that changed to regular Tylenol. She replied that she would check with Dr. Harkness.

She returned in about five minutes and said that Dr. Harkness would be here in a few minutes to talk with me but that the regular Tylenol would be okay. My family walked in as the nurse left the room. We sat and talked for a while. Then Dr. Harkness entered the room. "Paul, good news. The clot that was in your heart is gone. You're going to be just fine. You'll need to stay in the hospital for a while to get you off the medication that is thinning your blood now and put you back on Coumadin and have it stabilize your blood with the right dosage. The reason you had so much pain in your left side is that when the medicine busted up the clot, it went to your spleen and lodged there. That caused all the pain you were feeling. That deteriorated. So I don't see any complications with your recovery, but I'm going to keep you here for a while to make sure everything is back to normal."

We talked for a few minutes and then Dr. Harkness left. The family and I talked about what had happened. My sister and her husband decided they were going home since everything was okay with me. I also asked Angie and Mom and Dad to go home. I wanted Angie to go home so she could take care of Daniel and Brianna. Mom and Dad looked too tired to be sitting around there looking at me when there was absolutely nothing wrong with me now. They all agreed they could use a good night's rest, so they went home.

The family wasn't gone very long when the telephone rang. The phone was built into the railing that rose up and down on the right side of the bed, so access to it was very easy. When I answered, to my surprise I immediately recognized the voice as being Dr. Wyne. He wanted to know how everything was going. I explained what had taken place and that everything looked good. We talked for a while. After I hung the phone up, I realized how concerned he really was for me as I thought about how unusual it was for him to call.

I didn't do much for the next three days, but I was feeling much stronger. Dr. Harkness informed me that I was to be moved from the critical floor to a regular bed on another floor. As time passed I got stronger.

By the fifth day, when daybreak came, I was walking the halls. Dr. Harkness had started me on Coumadin the day before and removed the IV, so I had no restrictions. I was in a room with two beds, but I was the only occupant at that time. It was getting extremely lonely with no one to talk to. My wife's brother-in-law, Jim, would stop by almost every day for and hour or so. Jim lived only a few minutes from the hospital. He knew that I enjoyed a good cold Pepsi, so he'd bring me a couple each day. He was a man that could always find something to talk about, and when he wanted to say what was on his mind, he did. I looked forward to Jim's visit. But after he left, there was very little to do. The nurses would come and go. The cleaning people and the people from the lab would talk for a while, but they had jobs to do.

By the sixth day, I had to find something to occupy my time. As I left my room to enter the hall, I noticed to my left there was a man standing at the end of the hall, looking out the window. The hall was about twelve feet wide. A very large window took up all the space at the end, with the exception of the space heaters underneath. As I looked out the window, the sky was so blue, I felt like I had just looked at that part of the world for the first time. Straight across, I could see a very large building about eight stories high. The building was about two stories higher than the window where I was standing. On top of the building sat a helicopter. I assumed that it belonged to the hospital. As the helicopter took off, the sun was shining so brightly the reflection off the blades almost blinded me for a few seconds. As I watched that large object turn into a small dot in the sky, I could only wonder where they were going.

To my right was an empty hallway. About eight doors down was the nurse's station. As I stood there, I recalled the two large chairs in my room equipped with footstools. I asked the man at the window if he would help me drag those chairs out into the hall so we could place them in front of that window, so we did.

I stayed in the hospital for another eight days. Not once did I see those chairs empty. I got to meet people from all walks of life. After that day, there was never a moment when I couldn't walk in the hall and find someone to talk with. When nurses made their rounds, they would push their carts down to those big chairs and start calling out names. Most of the time, we sat in the floor and talked until someone gave up his or her chair or footstool.

It was about eleven o'clock one night. I was sitting in one of those chairs, watching the rainfall outside. As I sat there, a woman in her sixties occupied the other chair. I could tell by her cough, she was the lady who occupied the room next to mine. Until now, I had never seen her out of bed. She was a heavy woman with streaks of gray in her hair, which was tied in a bun on top. She introduced herself as Maxie May. As she talked, I realized how much she enjoyed talking about her family. She had a bright glow about her. In between the cough, she was smiling as she talked. To me, her enjoyment of life was beyond compare. We sat, watched the rain, and talked until the early hours of morning. After that, I would see Maxie May sitting in one of those chairs talking to someone each day, if only for a few minutes. She was still there with little change in her condition when I left.

Time passed. I was released from the hospital on Monday. I was asked to schedule an appointment with Dr. Wyne in two weeks for a checkup and return to Dr. Harkness' office in six months.

DISABILITY

I returned to my work a couple of days after my release. As I began to work, I felt a slight tightness in my chest. I began to realize that I was not in perfect health. From this day forward, I should set aside all the things I wanted to do with my life and devote all of my energy to the needs of my family.

In the past, I had done what I enjoyed as far as work was concerned, in hope of someday being successful. Now I realized that my health would not allow me to do that. I quit work until I would see Dr. Wyne in two weeks. I would ask him about Social Security Disability income.

Two weeks passed. I was sitting in an exam room waiting for Dr. Wyne. As he entered the room, he had a big smile on his face. When he shook my hand, he said, "Mr. Robinson, I was worried about you. When I saw you last, your chances of living weren't very good at all. I even called Duke University, to talk with an expert. Your future didn't look good, but I am glad to see you. I would like for you to go over to the hospital for another echocardiogram."

I agreed. Then I explained to him about the tightness in my chest when I started back to work and that I was short of breathe when carrying heavy objects. He asked the nurse to do an EKG there in the office. After that, I went to the hospital for the echocardiogram. After returning to Dr. Wyne's office, he informed me not to lift more than ten to fifteen pounds, not to push a lawnmower, and to stay away from stress or things that might upset me.

I asked Dr. Wyne about Social Security Disability income. He told me that his office would do everything possible to help me live a long life. If I needed anything, all I needed to do was to call.

The next day, I went to the Social Security office and gave them the necessary information to sign up for disability income. After the lady finished, I asked what Social Security benefits I would receive if I were found to be disabled. She explained that I would receive a monthly check of $850. After a six-month waiting period, I would receive a card.

I knew this wasn't going to be easy. Six months without financial income. I've heard talk that some people waited for two years.

A month had passed, and the bank was calling about my truck payment. I explained my condition to the man on the phone and told him there wasn't any money for a truck payment. He asked if I could bring the truck down to the bank in the next couple of days.

The next day, Angie followed me down to the bank. I felt that was the longest six miles I had ever traveled. My truck was important to me, but it was a small sacrifice. Trying to keep this truck was not in the best interest of my family.

Angie kept her car because of the disability insurance. Daniel, Brianna, and I needed a vehicle to ride while Angie was at work. I bought a 1975 Toyota Celica for $400.00 from a college student. The old car wasn't much, but it got the kids and me where we needed to go.

I had a little lumber left over from the business, so the kids and I built a deck on the front of our double wide. We would only work a couple of hours a day. Doing this gave us something to pass the time.

The days of summer were coming to an end. It was September and Daniel and Brianna had gone back to school. I would head for the mountains hunting ginseng. Digging ginseng (a wild herb) in the fall and selling the ginseng in December would make sure we would have Christmas money.

It was the last of October; the plants would be dying soon and the season coming to an end. Now I was finding it difficult to get out of bed in the morning. My days were long and lonely.

Angie was giving me twenty-five dollars a week for gas. The rest of her paycheck went for food and the house payment. This would be the first time in my life that I was unable to help with my family's financial problems. Believe me, I was feeling lower that a sole on a shoe.

We traveled once a month down to Kentucky to visit our family. They would give us boxes of food and a little gas money for traveling. I began to learn how to cook so that I could prepare the meals. After a while, my cooking became a problem—not with my family but with me. I had gained fourteen pounds in six months. My middle was spreading, and for some unknown reason I didn't seem to notice. I now weighed 190 pounds.

I went to see Dr. Wyne for my six-month check up. I was having chest pains about once a week that lasted for only five or ten seconds. Dr. Wyne said, "The test didn't show anything that would cause the pain, but I am concerned with your weight. The extra weight will put a serious strain on your heart. I would recommend a diet. The nurse will give you a diet sheet to go by, and you should also walk at least three miles a day."

A few days later, I received a letter from the social security office that I was rejected for disability income.

Winter had been difficult for me after my first operation. When temperatures drop below forty, I don't like being outside. Breathing cold air hurts my chest. Snow was in the air; my appeal for social security would take another six months or longer. I'd be stuck in the house for the winter. I was beginning to doubt my decision and myself as a man. I wondered what purpose I served in this life. Then I would remind myself of the promise I made to myself and to my family.

Winter of 1992-93 was difficult, to say the least. During the summer of 1993, nothing had changed with my life, except my ability to cook. That has only gotten better. My middle had gotten bigger. I now weighed 195 pounds. I knew what I should do, but I have difficult keeping my sanity. I had learned what being lonely is. It's a horrible thing.

We were still visiting our family in Kentucky. Daniel and I were going down to the river fishing when we had gas money. Angie took a second job cleaning the building where she worked.

It was midsummer and another letter of rejection had arrived. I decided to appeal again-only this time with a lawyer. Summer was gone. The dreaded months of winter were upon me again. I must keep my sanity. Dr. Wyne was getting extremely worried about me. I now weighed 205 pounds. I knew my weight was a problem but I couldn't control it.

Dr. Wyne made a statement that I should always be there for my family and the only way to do that is to keep your body in the best physical conditions possible. I suddenly realized I was slowly destroying the most precious thing in my life by eating. My heart never gave up on me. Perhaps somewhere hidden deep in my mind, I thought that because my heart was damaged then repaired, I would never be the man I was before the operation. The only part of my body that had been damaged was my mind. I decided, "If my heart can carry an extra twenty-nine pounds of fat and perform to the highest standard of quality, then I shall lose the fat and let my heart be free so that I may live up to my highest standard of quality as a man."

It's spring of 1994. I have another problem, or should I say a war made up of battles that I would fight and win each day for the rest of my life. Before I was hospitalized in 1992, I was smoking two packs of cigarettes a day as I had been for the past seven years. While I was lying in the hospital, I was thinking of cigarettes a lot and how I wished I could have one draw. Then I asked myself why I smoked. Was it because I enjoy getting up in the morning, going to the bathroom and spitting for thirty minutes trying to clear my lungs? Maybe it was coughing for the next two hours or maybe it was the sniffing, snorting and people asking if I was sick, or perhaps the smell on my clothes. After all of that, I decided cigarettes were nothing more than a habit that was damaging my health. Quitting cold turkey was easy. I realized that my eating problem was nothing more than a habit, but I can't quit eating so I must learn how to eat.

Four months had passed. I wasn't doing well with my eating problem. I was still suffering from depression, mostly because there was no money. The mortgage company was calling about our loan on the double wide. I had fought my eating problem to where I was at a peak with my weight. I was averaging between 200 and 205 pounds. I felt that was a step in the right direction, and I wasn't giving up.

I received a letter informing me of a court hearing scheduled in August for Social Security. As the day of our salvation arrived, Angie, Daniel, Brianna and I packed a lunch—"coal miners steak sandwiches", which were bologna sandwiches. The hearing was scheduled on a Tuesday at eleven a.m. our trip was a one and half-hour drive. We left three hours early. When the hearing was over and we left the courtroom, we thought judgment was in our favor, but we still had to wait for the judge's decision.

About two weeks later, we received a letter stating that our Social Security was approved. We had plans to treat ourselves to a night out on the town and a large steak dinner. By the time our first check came in September, the excitement had slowed down. We had taught ourselves to be conservative—going out would be a waste of money. We ended up going to the grocery and having a large steak dinner at home.

Angie decided to continue with her second job. There were so many things we had to do without over the past two years. We needed to catch up on unpaid bills and buy new clothes, among other things.

STOPPING THE PAIN

Its September—ginseng season is here again. I now brought home a check, which I felt better about, but I was still fighting depression. Ginseng hunting keeps me busy through October. Angie told me of an exercise club in Blacksburg that was only a twenty-minute drive from home. I could not imagine lifting a piece of iron or standing in one place running unless someone paid me to, but I was determined to lose the weight, so I decided to give it a try.

As I entered the club, all I could see was a lot of equipment that I didn't know the first thing about. I stood there wondering why people would work so hard at doing nothing until I looked down at my stomach. I asked the young lady behind the desk about an exercise program that would help me lose weight. She began to explain that I could sign up for one month for twenty-five dollars. With that I got three free sessions with a professional trainer. I signed up because the mention of a trainer peaked my interest. I also needed help.

The next morning, I arrived in my shorts and a tee shirt, ready for my first session. I could do this. I've been ginseng hunting in mountains and working around the house. I am over weight but I think I am in fairly good condition. My trainer was a young man in his early twenties, around six-feet tall, nothing but muscle and blood. I thought, "If I look half that good, Angie would have a new man."

My first lesson was the treadmill. He explained that this machine would help me lose weight and build up strength in my heart muscle. He explained how the machine worked, and then he set my pace at 2.5, which was a very slow walk. He set the timer for a thirty-minute walk. As he walked away, I notice a woman with streaks of gray in her hair, maybe in her sixties, on the machine next to mine. Her pace was set at 3.5.

I knew this was embarrassing, but I decided on my first day, I should do as the instructor asked. There was a big screen TV to watch. It was a slow steady walk. I could do this all day. When the thirty minutes was over, the machine had a five-minute cool down period. I remember the instructor telling me to make sure to do the cool down, so I did. When the machine stopped, I was going to jump off and go up front to ask the instructor what was next. As I turned to get off the machine, my head started to spin. Then I fell flat in the floor. As I started to get up, the lady with

45

the streaks of gray in her hair grabbed my hand to help me up and asked, "Are you all right young man?" That was embarrassing.

I sat on the treadmill for a few minutes to collect myself. I decided that was enough for one day.

For the next two weeks, I sat at home because I was ashamed of my condition and too embarrassed to go back, knowing that everyone would be looking at me, laughing because I had fallen. Feeling sorry for myself wasn't going to help, so on my next trip back to the club, I checked in at the front desk, turned and went straight to the treadmill and began to walk. No one paid any attention. It was like I had never been there. I walked for thirty minutes at 2.5. When my time was over, I got off very slowly.

I only attended the club a couple of times a week during the winter. I could never really feel comfortable. The only time that I ever felt the need to walk was when I didn't have a ride.

When Angie and I were first married, I made a promise to build her a new home—a promise that I wasn't able to keep until now. With the back pay from social security and a lot of luck, we could take our money and buy land, and then sell our doublewide. Our problem was finding land in our price range of fifteen thousand. About six months had passed. We finally located a piece of land along the foothills of Clover Hollow Mountain. There laid eight acres, full of red oak, maple, and poplar trees. A small stream trickles through the tall timber. It's a beautiful place we began to call home.

In the spring of 1995, we began cutting brush and clearing the land for our new home. We were waiting in hopes of making a profit from the sale of our doublewide so that money could go toward having the well and septic put in.

Summer has passed. I had forgotten about walking, but I was trying to watch now much I ate. I convinced myself that when I traveled anywhere, if I could pass up a store or a fast food restaurant I would be able to lose weight. It worked. Just by doing that one simple task, I lost five pounds over the summer. I knew that wasn't much, but that was five pounds that I felt good about. I now weighed between 195 and 200 pounds.

That's not to say I never eat out because I do when someone is with me. If they want to stop, I will have something to eat, but while traveling alone, I will not stop and eat.

During the last week in September, we accepted an offer on our doublewide trailer. We had until the first week in December to move. On our new property, Daniel and I were building a temporary structure to live in. Also during this time, we were having the well and septic put in. Angie and Brianna, in their spare time, were packing boxes and cleaning the doublewide. Moving was a lot of hard work, but as we pulled together as a family, we moved to our new home first week in December, as scheduled.

The winter of 1995/96 was colder than normal. Snow had begun to fall a few days after we moved in. The temporary structure that Daniel and I built was incomplete; our building was only twenty-four feet square. We angled the roof high enough for two small bedrooms upstairs. The insulation was the only thing between the outer walls and us. We put up quilts for inside doors. A wood burning stove, which was our main source of heat, took up most of the space in the living room. We were stuck in this house most of the winter. Because of the amount of snow we had to contend with and our finances, we couldn't build until the spring of 1997.

During the summer of 1996, Daniel and I worked around the house. Brianna got a job, which kept her busy. On the weekends, we all pitched in to help Angie with her second job.

I have realized that controlling not what I eat but how much I eat is my biggest problem. I love to eat. I was so bad that thirty minutes after lunch, I could walk into the kitchen and my body would tell me that I was hungry or at least that's what I thought—another habit that was very difficult to break.

I began to keep a notebook of how much food I ate per day; I even kept down what and how much I drank. On any given day that I felt bad, I would go back and check my notes and realize the amount of food I ate the day before was probably causing my discomfort. I was eating enough for two people to survive; my eating habits were so routine that my body would fight me if I varied from my eating schedule at all. For instance, my head or my stomach would hurt until I ate something. Day after day I would go a little longer, until one day I was only eating three meals a day, nothing in between. My only problem now was eating after supper while sitting and watching T.V. And eating late was a big habit. My weight was averaging between 190 and 195 by the end of summer.

During the winter of 1996-97 we were comfortable living in our temporary home. Because our finances were in order, I began working with the bank on loaning us the money to build our new home. I also started walking at the weight club in hopes of setting aside the depression I get each winter. In March our loan came through. The process took longer than we thought, but I insisted on being my own contractor; by doing that we estimated a large savings. My depression only lasted about twenty days during the winter; that wasn't too bad. I was feeling better with each day that passed. Chest pains that lasted five or ten seconds were occurring around once a month. Sometimes I didn't remember if the pain occurred the month before or not. I was doing two to four miles a day walking. My weight was now averaging from185 to 190.

I gave up walking in April when construction began on our new house. Daniel and I were doing all the light work to the house. When the framing started, we hired contractors to finish the job.

During the summer, I tried to control how much I ate, but my main concern was finishing our house. On September 1st, one promise came true. We moved into our new home. Angie's dream had become a reality.

It was also time for another check up with doctor Wyne. I had a problem with my cholesterol. When my weight reached 205, my cholesterol was 331. Now my weight was 187 and my cholesterol had dropped to 261. Dr. Wyne was pleased and so was I.

I believe that I can fulfill my promise by March 1998. By dedicating myself to a light excerise program and watching how much I eat, losing ten pounds should not be a problem.

Thanksgiving and Christmas would be here soon. Angie insists on fixing dinner for both holidays including all her pies and cakes. We also went to Kentucky this time of year. We averaged a week for each holiday, and everyone we visit, insisted that we have a meal and dessert before leaving. These meals were southern cooking. They don't believe that a sandwich, pop and chips were a meal. Nooo! We're looking at fried chicken, green beans, fried taters, and cole slaw, corn bread and to top this meal off, we're looking at maybe apple pie with ice cream or stack cake with coffee. These meals are fixed twice a day during the holidays and for breakfast—buttermilk biscuit; gravy made from sausage grease, eggs, bacon, and sausage and fried taters. These meals were needed when I was growing up, because everyone was doing manual labor from sunrise to sunset. The days of hard labor are gone but not forgotten. I think my chances of moving a mountain would be easier than losing weight during the holidays.

I felt that losing weight was very important to me, but being in the best physical condition possible should also be my ultimate goal.

I began by joining the weight club again. The club had a new set of scales for weighing yourself. These scales weighed in ounces, which I enjoyed very much. On my first day I weighed in at 187.6. I considered myself eleven pounds over weight.

I began by getting on the treadmill. I set the speed at 3.5, which was a comfortable walk. I could feel the fat in my stomach and chest going up and down with each step. It felt horrible. On my first day I only walked a mile. When I finished, I weighed myself. I had lost four ounces. Was it fat or was it water that I lost? I didn't care—it was four ounces. I liked that. If I hadn't been so tired, I would have walked another mile.

After my first month, I was walking between two and three miles a day. After about six weeks, I began to jog a little. With each walk, not much maybe one half mile, I was feeling good. I was watching how much I ate. My weight was at 185.

Thanksgiving and Christmas have come and gone. I did indulge on all the wonderful food, but not as much as in the past holidays. With each day when I had the opportunity and sometimes when I didn't, I would slip away to the weight club. I knew if I didn't go the extra mile, my promise would not be kept.

January 1998, it was time to see Dr. Wyne. I knew I was doing well. By this time I was jogging; not walking, but jogging, between two and four miles a day and watching how much I was eating, I didn't remember the last time I felt pain of any kind. I was feeling good. Nothing could go wrong.

Each time before I visited Doctor Wyne, I would go and have my blood drawn so he could tell me the results during my visit. You know when you visit the doctor's office, the nurse takes you in and the first thing she says is, "Hop up on these scales. Let's see how much you weigh." Hey, I was ready. No more, "Oh, Adam you put on some pounds!" This time she said, "Adam you lost five pounds since your last visit." I was smiling from ear to ear. Then she went and burst my bubble. She said, "Adam your blood work shows that your cholesterol has gone from 261 back up to 331. Doctor Wyne will discuss this with you."

Dr. Wyne said that I was looking good but he couldn't understand why my cholesterol would jump seventy points in just six months. He also put me on cholesterol medication and instructed me to have my cholesterol checked in two months. By the time I got home I was really aggravated. I hated the thought of taking any kind of medication so I began to read everything I could find on cholesterol and the foods that are high in cholesterol. After doing this, I began to realize that all those holidays cakes and pies, and all that southern cooking that was made with so much love was about to kill me.

I began to make a list of all the foods that were high in cholesterol so that I could eliminate those foods from my diet, or at least work hard at it. I decided I would also talk with an exercise instructor in the near future to make sure that I was doing my exercises correctly and ask them to show me an exercise within my guidelines that would help increase my upper body strength.

March 19, 1998—the moment of truth. I had learned the hard way that even though I can lose weight by watching how much I eat, foods that are high in cholesterol are just as bad for me as being thirty pounds overweight. My weight is 174 and my cholesterol at 161.

GETTING A LIFE

May 1998. I received a letter from Social Security, stating that it was time to reevaluate my disability. In the letter they explained that I was to see a psychiatrist in August.

I had been on disability income since 1992. I had found life easy as far as doing things physically; but as for my mental state, life on disability income was one that I found very difficult. I felt my only contribution in life was taking up space and depleting the world of oxygen. I existed to watch others as they went about their life. I truly missed being part of that world.

I wanted to return to work and be a part of the world around me but I was scared. During the winter months I found it difficult to breathe when the weather got below forty degrees outside. I knew I had to look for a job indoors.

August, I visited with the psychiatrist. My session was about thirty minutes, but I was so scared, the session felt like just five minutes long.

I put on a good show. I walked around the office and smiled, answered his questions with energy to spare. When I was walking to my car, I realized the answers I gave put me back into the work force where I wanted to be. In October I received a letter from Social Security stating that they found me mentally and physically capable of returning to work and to reapply for SS benefits I should do so before I received the last check, which would be in January 1999.

The next morning I was off to the employment office. I had to find something indoors. After two weeks of looking through the newspapers and applying for jobs that I was not qualified for, I was beginning to think of reapplying for Social Security.

A friend of mine from Virginia Tech who knew my circumstances called and told me about a program he was starting at Tech, and he offered me a job. I began work in January of 1999. My office was a five by six with a window, a desk and a computer. I would spend the next fourteen months in this office. Rising from my sleep at six each morning, going to the gym and working out for an hour, working in this office for eight hours, and trying to watch how much I ate was a very difficult job. For fourteen months I had held steady and my weight was still the same. The program at Tech had ended and I was back looking for a job again.

It was the middle of summer and I was building and selling outdoor furniture for extra money while looking for a job. My wife called and told me she saw a help wanted ad in the paper. A person who I had sold firewood to about six years previous was now operating a private facility called Tekoa that housed and schooled young teenage females in Floyd, Virginia. She was looking for an administrative assistant. I was not qualified to be an administrate assistance, but I called to apply. Susan Sisk explained that the position had been filled but she had another position opened for a part time maintenance man if I would be interested.

I took the job and started in September of 2000—two days a week, ten hours a day. That was good. I could continue building and selling furniture. I was back doing what I enjoyed most—working with my hands and being outside in the fresh air. I hoped to never be restricted to an office job again.

With my new job, I was down to visiting the gym only two days a week, but I was still holding steady with my weight.

By April of 2001, Tekoa started another facility for boys in Christiansburg, Virginia, which increased my position to full time.

GAINING WEIGHT

Working fulltime had become a problem for me. It was not like it was when I was staying at home. I had been going to the gym everyday, coming back home, eating the foods that I wanted to fix, resting when I got tired, and taking life easy.

Working four days a week, ten hours a day as a maintenance man, I was on my feet all day but not really getting any exercise. I was simply walking from one job to another. Then I had the problem with food; up at 5:30am each morning, always in a hurry for work, grabbing breakfast on the road usually at a fast food restaurant. Snacks were whatever I could find. Lunch was a fast food restaurant or at the facility where I was working and I usually had an afternoon snack. By the time I got home around 6:00 each evening, I was averaging a twelve-hour day. Angie would get home before I did and would have supper ready when I got there. Each evening I would eat too much because I was so hungry, then sit in my favorite chair relaxing because I felt so exhausted from the day. I would watch TV till eight or nine o'clock. Then I would find something to eat, not from hunger, mostly from boredom. Then I'd go to bed.

Over the winter months I suffered from depression again. I weighed 184 pounds. I could feel the fat in a large roll around my stomach. I would find it very difficult to walk because my left knee hurt when I walked any distance at all, and my days of running were gone.

Something had to change. I was not allowing myself to get fat again.

As a maintenance man, my job was to assess the problem, figure out what it takes to fix the problem, and then get the job done. I now felt I had a major problem with my eating. I decided the first thing to do was to have my eating problem as my number one priority in my life, above all others. This includes my job, my wife, my children and the rest of my family. I knew I wasn't the only person that lived with heart disease. My wife, my children, my mom, dad and the rest of the family live with it also. When I got overweight, I could see the worry in their eyes; wondering, "Is Adam physically capable of doing things? Will he have a heart attack?" I didn't want that. I wanted everyone to look at me as a person who was capable of doing everyday living, without someone worrying about me.

I was forty-six years of age, and I understood that blockage in the arteries at my age was very likely, especially with the type of food that I was eating and the fact that I was overweight. I had gone through one open-heart surgery. Whatever it would take to keep myself healthy, I would do it.

My first step was to figure out how much food I was eating, what type of food I was eating, and how to cut back. I created my own personal diet program because I wasn't capable of following those so-called diets that are on the market today. My program would be for the rest of my life.

MY HEALTH PROGRAM

First step: Learn to think positively! Think of how much food I'm eating every-day and how to cut back on my food intake. This step alone will be my most difficult.

Second Step: Implement an exercise program that enables me to learn to do simple exercise, strengthen the heart muscle and tighten the loose skin from the weight I'm going to lose.

Third Step: Learn about different foods, how food affects my body, how to count calories, what foods I should be eating and what foods I should not be eating.

This program will help me feel better, look better, and have more confidence. In return I will help others—my family and friends.

What do I want?

I want to lose weight, of course, look physically fit, and feel good every morning when I get up.

Think positively! I must convince myself that I really want to lose the weight. Think of how I want to look and feel next year, five years or ten years from today. I must realize what one person can do, another can do.

This program is very simple: to teach myself how to cut back on the amount of food I put into my body.

What will I accomplish?

I will learn how to cut back on my food intake, learn to exercise, learn what foods are good for me and the food that makes me gain weight. What I learn I must practice every day for the rest of my life.

I eat at certain times during the day. I have a schedule, that's a habit.

I feel that my mind and body are separate. My mind controls my body. My mind has created an eating habit for my body. My body recognizes these eating habits during different times of the day.

I will recognize those habits and begin to change those habits one at a time. This will be very difficult because once I begin to change my habits; my body will recognize these changes. My body will feel discomfort or on edge. My stomach may start to swell. I may feel sick on my stomach or get a headache. All of this will pass.

Communication in my house will be very important. I will explain to Angie about my program, and what I'm trying to accomplish, and that I will need her support and help.

My first step is to eliminate all the temptation in my home such as cookies, cakes, candy, ice cream, peanut butter, cold cuts, leftovers, bread, etc.—anything that's quick and easy to fix. Replace these items with apples, oranges, and other healthy choices until I learn to control my cravings.

There will be no food three hours before bedtime or during the night. I know this will be very difficult to accomplish, but there are tricks to help myself.

- Trick #1: Buy myself about thirty packs of chewing gum. When I want that late night snack, I'll grab a pack of gum.

- Trick #2: Go to bed one hour early.

- Trick #3: When I can't take the pressure for three hours, and I must have something to eat, I'll try apples, oranges, grapes or any type of fruit.

Angie and I will pick one evening a week that we choose a late snack. Friday or Saturday will be the best. Make this snack something special for us, and make sure we don't overdo it. Example: If we had cake and ice cream and had a good serving, we will not save the remainder but throw it out. If it's left in the house someone will eat it, and most likely, it will be me, so we will throw it out.

As an overeater I need to keep records of my daily eating and exercise activities. I created these eighteen forms for me to fill out daily. At the top of each page I have incentives to remind me of how important this program is for me. I will be able to answer my own question's like, how much food did I consume today, was the food healthy for me, did I get enough exercise today?

DAY—ONE
WHAT I PRACTICE,
THOSE AROUND ME WILL PRACTICE

NAME		DAY	DATE	COUNT CALORIE
	WHAT DID I EAT?		WHERE DID I EAT	
BREAKFAST 7:00AM 9:00AM				
SNACK 10:30AM				
LUNCH BETWEEN 12:00PM & 2:00PM				
SNACK 3:30PM				
SUPPER BETWEEN 5:00PM & 7:00PM				
EATING AFTER HOURS	HOW MUCH DID I EAT TODAY	WWW.NUTRITIOND ATA.COM		TOTAL

DID I EXERCISE TODAY? EXPLAIN.

DAY—TWO
I MUST REALIZE HOW MUCH FOOD I'M EATING

DAY—THREE
ALL YOU CAN EAT BUFFET.
MAKE SURE I GET MY MONEY'S WORTH.
GAIN FIVE POUNDS.

DAY—FOUR
I CAN LOSE THE WEIGHT.
TODAY IS A NEW DAY.

DAY—FIVE
DON'T EAT AFTER 7:00 PM.
GET A COMFORTABLE NIGHT'S SLEEP.
GET A FULL NIGHT'S SLEEP.

DAY—SIX
WHAT DO I WANT?
STAY STRONG.
STAY FOCUSED.

DAY—SEVEN
EVERYTHING I DO TAKES EFFORT,
NO MATTER WHAT I DO.

DAY—EIGHT
EATING HABITS I CREATE WITH THIS PROGRAM
I WILL PRACTICE FOR THE REST OF MY LIFE.

DAY—NINE
DID I DRINK ENOUGH WATER TODAY
EIGHT GLASSES A DAY

DAY—TEN
I'M PROUD OF MYSELF.
I AM DOING GREAT.

DAY—ELEVEN
FEEL GREAT.
EAT LESS.

DAY—TWELVE
GOING OUT FOR DINNER?
I'LL ASK MY SERVER
NOT TO SERVE BREAD
UNTIL THE MEAL IS SERVED.

DAY—THIRTEEN
FRUITS AND VEGETABLES-
FIVE PER-DAY.

DAY—FOURTEEN
BE HONEST TO MYSELF.
KEEP GOOD RECORDS.
UNDERSTAND MY HABITS.

DAY—FIFTEEN
THE POUNDS WILL SNEAK UP ON ME.
WATCH MY WEIGHT EVERYDAY.
DON'T OVEREAT.

DAY—SIXTEEN
HOW DO I WANT TO LOOK AND FEEL
ONE YEAR FROM TODAY?
TEN YEARS FROM TODAY?
DON'T OVEREAT.

DAY—SEVENTEEN
RESIST THE TEMPTATION.
EAT ONLY WHEN I'M HUNGRY.
I CAN LOSE THE WEIGHT.

DAY—EIGHTEEN
PARENTS ARE THE GREATEST TEACHERS ON EARTH
I'LL TEACH MY CHILDREN GOOD EATING HABITS
DON'T OVEREAT

WHAT I LEARNED IN EIGHTEEN DAYS.

I found out that working fulltime and trying to exercise and lose weight at the same time was a very difficult job. Though I had done two or three jobs simultaneously, I had found that trying to concentrate on exercise and losing weight while working ten hours a day was more difficult than I expected.

I had to convince Angie that I was very serious about this program. Angie only halfway believed me until a couple of days into the program.

A young man from up the road came riding his bike up my drive way and asked, "Adam would you go riding with me?"

Matt was sixteen, a nice looking young man. He stood about five feet seven inches tall, with dark hair and a very muscular built. I didn't know if Matt was serious or not, because he knew I wasn't physically capable of riding a bike to his ability. I expected that none of his friends lived within bike riding distance of him, and I was the only person he could think of to go bike riding.

"Sure, Matt, I'll go with you," I said.

I had a bad left knee and was looking for something to offset my walking, and maybe riding a bike was the answer.

I went in and told Angie where we were going, and she just put on that sneaky little grin and said okay. I knew what she was thinking; maybe he will go and maybe he won't.

I live on a dirt road about one quarter mile from the highway. I grabbed my son's bike that he left here when he went off to college. Matt and I put our bikes in the back of the old pickup and headed for the highway.

Matt had a gadget on his bike that marked off the miles as we rode our bikes. Six miles was the best I could do that day.

The next day I was so sore, but I enjoyed the ride very much, and riding the bicycle was the alternative to keeping my knee from hurting. I was getting the exercise I wanted.

The next evening, Matt and I rode again. After working ten hours, riding a bike any distance was extremely difficult. I really didn't think I was going to make this exercise work for me. The muscles I didn't even know existed in my body hurt so badly that I was barely able to walk from the truck into the house. When I came through the back door, Angie was taking everything out of the kitchen cabinets that was junk food or easy-to-fix foods. She grinned and said, "If you can do this I can too." I knew I was doing something right.

CUTTING BACK

I have said many times that you've got to eat. Unlike a cigarette habit, where you can quit cold turkey, one must eat. That's true. A person must eat, but I quit eating. I did. I quit eating. I quit eating at fast food restaurants. I quit eating at all-you-can-eat buffets. I quit eating pizza. I quit eating salt. I quit eating lots of food. Today, I live healthier, stronger, and I know that I am physically fit.

MEATS

For the past few years, most of the time after a meal, I had a knot in the top of my stomach. After a couple of hours, that knot would relax, then go away. I was worried so I went and saw the family doctor. She sent me to a specialist. After a few tests, he found nothing and suggested more serious testing. I told him I would think about it.

After the first week into the program, keeping records made me realize how much meat I was eating. I loved chicken, hamburgers and sausage. I didn't like the idea of eating so much protein, because I had read that meat was high in cholesterol. I had been fighting high cholesterol and taking medication for a very long time. Because of this program, I realized what I was doing to myself. Now, I only eat sausage and hamburgers maybe once a month, but chicken I still eat daily, only in smaller portions. The knot that was causing me so much trouble was not because of the meat I was eating but how much meat I was putting in my stomach on a daily basis.

WATER

I also realized that although I was substituting water for Pepsi when I was thirsty, especially when I stopped for gas, I still thought I needed a snack.

I decided to start bringing a bottle of water from home, so that when I stop for gas, I could go directly to the cashier. I wouldn't look left or right, only directly at the casher. I'll walk straight in, pay for the gas, and then get back out as quickly as possible. And the snacking, I just quit that.

I only drink three things: water, orange juice and Pepsi. The only time I drink Pepsi now, is when I have lunch and supper, and then only around four ounces, because I realize that too much is not a good thing. I drink orange juice only during the morning with breakfast, and even then, only one glass. Now when I'm thirsty, I only drink water. I try to drink my eight glasses of water per day, but that's a very difficult task, especially in the winter months.

My physical activity also slows down during the winter months, and some days I have to force myself to remember to drink water. I'll get a pack of teaberry chewing gum, and mixing the flavor of the gum with water as I chew. I'm able to drink around thirty-two ounces of bottled water in a short period of time. From April through October, I'll drink a lot of water because the days of summer are longer. My activities make me sweat, and I like drinking a lot of water when I sweat.

EATING OUT

When I was growing up, once a month or when Mom and Dad had the extra money, they would gather up the family on a Saturday evening and give us a taste of different food, something besides vegetables, soup beans and hog meat. There were five kids in the family, and we all piled into the back of the old Ford pickup. If the truck started, we headed downtown to the one and only fast food restaurant, Flannerys, better known to everyone in the neighborhood as The Greasy Spoon. At The Greasy Spoon, Dad would order chili-slaw burgers, an order of fries and an RC Cola for everyone. Mom would let down the tailgate of the truck, and we all sat in the back enjoying our treat. For dessert, we all got our favorite ice cream cone.

The food we were eating from the garden when I was growing up was the best food money could buy. I didn't realize it then, but I do now. Today I don't believe the fast food restaurants are any different than they were in yesteryear. There are just more of them. They are still the same old greasy spoons—better names and pretty buildings, but still just greasy spoons.

I watch families at fast food restaurants place their orders—nothing but meat and fries. The kids order the same size sandwich and fries their parents do.

As a heart patient of twenty years, and knowing what I know now, eating at a fast food restaurant more than once a week will do nothing for me except clog my arteries, make me fat, and keep me fat. What I decided to do is to quit eating any fast food—like smoking, just simply stop. Now the only time I eat at any fast food restaurant is when a group of people goes out to lunch or when one of my children asks to eat lunch and they decide where to go.

ALL-YOU-CAN-EAT BUFFET

I used to think this was the place to have a good meal, but as an overeater and a heart patient, I realized I was just hurting myself. Going into one of these places was like being ten years old again, with a dollar in my hand in a candy store. (That would be in the year 1965 when candy bars were only a nickel.) An all-you-can-eat buffet is nothing more than a hog feeder. Pay your eight or nine dollars and eat any kind of food you can think of—all you can stuff in your stomach for as long as you can eat. When I used to eat at these places, I would go by a table and see children with two or three plates. Today I stay away from these places except going out with a group of people or a co-worker or something of that nature. That doesn't happen very often, maybe a couple of times a year.

WINTER TIME DEPRESSION

I have fought winter time depression most of my adult life—never very serious depression, just sitting around not wanting to do anything, giving short answers, easily aggravated, small stuff like that. The past four years, I have suffered very little, if any, because of working with my program. I have figured out the cause of my depression. My depression usually starts around the last of October and lasts on and off through December. The answer is sugar. I've never had a problem with sugar physically, but I will admit I am addicted to it. I fight that addiction daily. If it's in my house, I will find it. I will even eat the jelly from the refrigerator just to taste the sugar. The last of October is Halloween. Candy is everywhere I go,—lying on peoples' desk and handed out at parades. The sugar is everywhere.

By the time I'm coming down from that high, it's Thanksgiving. Thanksgiving starts around the middle of November with lots of office parties and the neighbors coming by with cookies. The sugar flows like a stream. By the middle of December, when I'm coming down from that high, it starts all over again with Christmas. By then, all the sugar is starting to get a little old, and by Christmas Day, I will eat very little. The day after Christmas, if there's any sugar left, we will give it away or throw it away. When New Year's Day has come, my depression has disappeared until next winter.

That is my wintertime depression that I have suffered with for so long. I didn't understand what was wrong until I started this program. I still suffer a little during these months, because I am an OVEREATER and sugar is my weakness.

January 17, 2005, almost four years since I started my program. Have I been true to the program? No, of course not. I'm still an OVEREATER, but I have worked at it every single day.

Maybe I will eat at a fast food restaurant. Maybe I will eat at an all-you-can-eat buffet. Maybe I will have a candy bar and a Pepsi. Maybe Angie and I will go out for dinner. Maybe, but that doesn't happen very often because I fight to stay healthy.

I still work at Tekoa, ten hours a day, Monday through Thursday. I go to the gym on the weekends when I'm not fishing, I still ride my bike during the summer months, after work and during weekends. I even did the Floyd Fifty, Mountain Parkway bike ride in 2004, and finished the ride in five and half hours.

I will celebrate my fiftieth birthday in March. I stand 5'9" tall, weigh 170 pounds, am physically fit, and I feeling very good about myself. I will continue to fight to keep my heart and body healthy for me and for the ones I love.

Conclusion

After twenty-five years of heart disease I have figured out that life is to short. Pain, stress, overweight, and these three health problems I have conquered. If I have pain in my body, I must have done something to cause the pain. Did I eat too much? Did I get enough sleep? If two Tylenol doesn't take care of the problem I'll see a doctor.

I will not allow stress to be a part of my life. My family may have a problem that causes me a little stress every once in a while. With time, patience, love and a lot of communication that problem is taken care of in a day or two. I go to work everyday and do a good job. It's the kind of work I like and a lot of communication between my employer and me and my co-workers helps eliminate any stress at work.

I still have dreams that I am fat. I'll wake up in the middle of the night with my heart racing and I'll feel of my stomach just to make sure that I'm not fat before I can go back to sleep.

I now walk or jog three to five miles a day, five days a week. I also do a light upper body exercise each day. I am consistent about doing one hour of exercise per day.

When I get up each morning, I look forward to going to the club. I don't think it's the club that I looked forward to. It's the sweat that rolls down the back of my neck and the deep breaths that I take while biking that clears my lungs. I believe that I will continue to exercise from this day forward, because I don't remember the last time that I had chest pain. I look physically fit, I feel great, and Angie runs me out of the house each morning because she can't cope with me—my energy level puts me in high gear.

If I could go back and change anything at all in my life that I wanted to, what would I change? Nothing! I have had a great life; sure I have had a few hard knocks, but I have had a great life, and I feel I'm only beginning to live. I have Angie to grow old with. I have two wonderful children, Daniel and Brianna and maybe if I'm lucky I'll have a few grandkids somewhere in the future. I also have my Mom and Dad and my brothers and sisters and a few good friends. What more could I want or need.

I give thanks everyday to God for my good fortune of health and happiness and that of my family.

Adam

978-0-595-35634-8
0-595-35634-6